tarts with

- Anna

't Let your Dreams

have no choice to be your advocate.

nk-tops lenecks

"Hello. It's Meh."

AF510828

But look at how far you've come.

Everyone wants happiness, no one wants pain, but you can't have a rainbow, without a little rain.

If only our tongues were made of glass, would we be more careful of what we said?

She love she

Okay?

Oka

#WIFI box

That's the thing about pain, it demands to be felt.

Once upon a time you were my everything

♡ I live my b

its me

I just need someone to LISTEN

And there was no way to avoid the cruelness of the spinning

you can build confidence once you free yourself of other people's judgements.

AN ORDINARY DAY

KIDS WITH RARE GENETIC CONDITIONS

KAREN HABERBERG

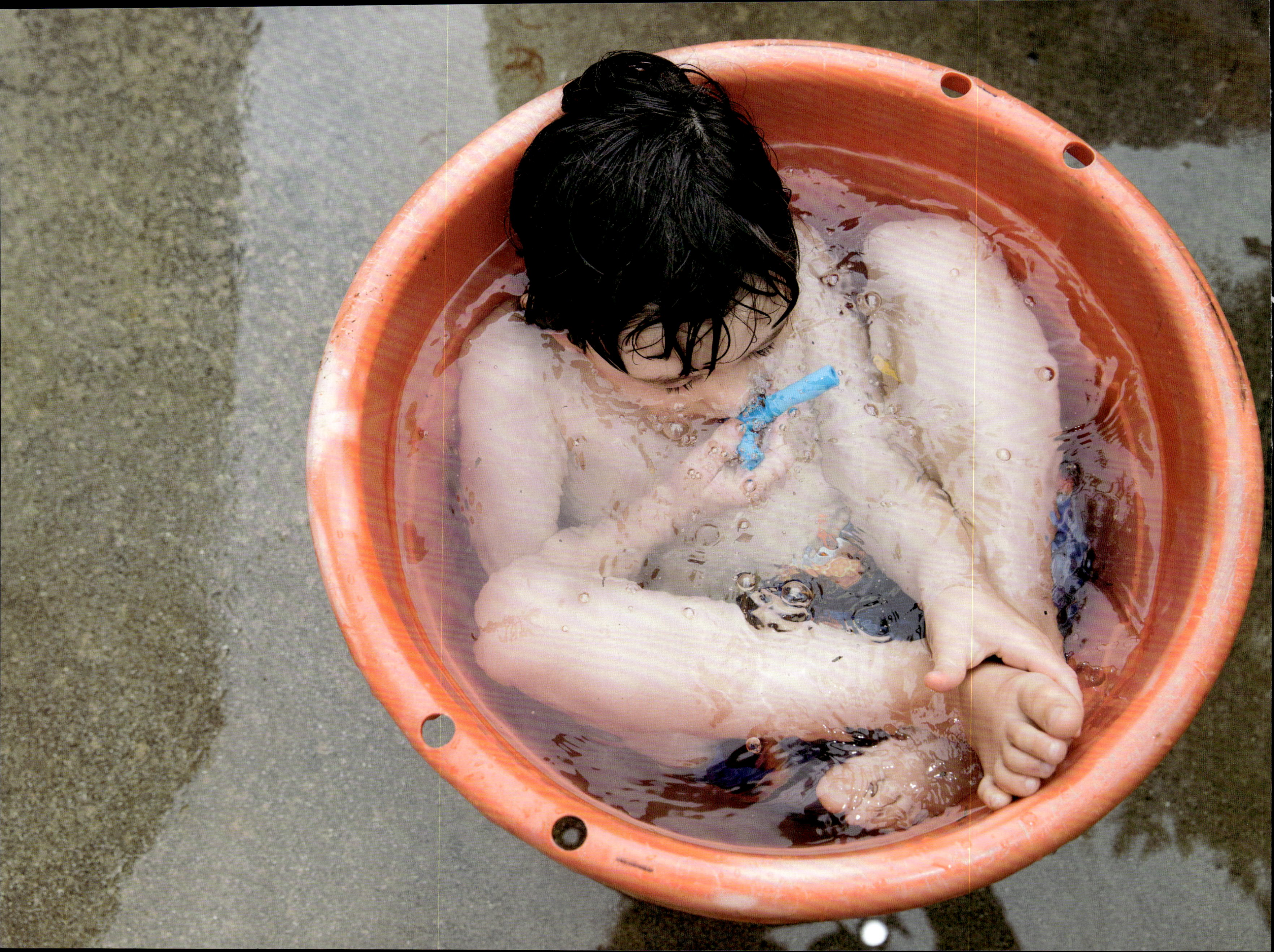

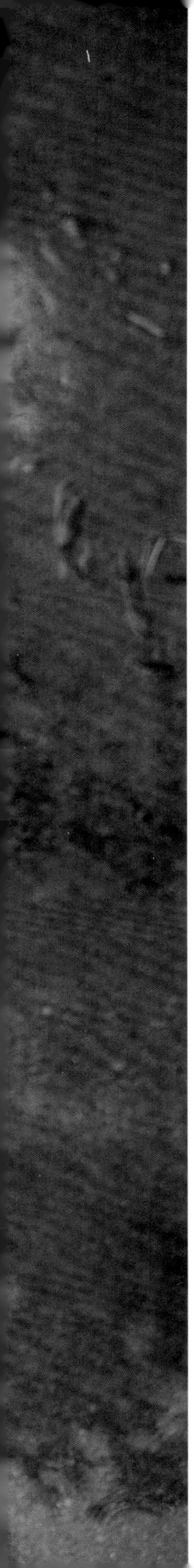

AN ORDINARY DAY: KIDS WITH RARE GENETIC CONDITIONS

KAREN HABERBERG

Photo Editor: Robert Peacock

powerHouse Books
Brooklyn, NY

Foreword

Severe genetic diseases are individually rare, but collectively common, affecting more than one in every twenty people in the U.S. These diseases carry with them a tremendous burden of human suffering, accounting for one tenth of all pediatric hospital admissions and up to a fifth of all infant deaths. In each of the families affected by these diseases, just one or two spelling changes among the three billion letters of DNA in a child's genome have led to an altered protein that affects the function of their body. These tiny genetic changes can affect any part of the body, with different diseases affecting the brain, lungs, liver, blood, bones, skin, or any other tissues—and forever changing the lives of patients, as well as those that love them.

Genetic diseases are testament to the complexity and fragility of the human body. We develop in the womb as a patchwork of tissues and cells of almost unimaginable precision, guided at each step by information encoded in the DNA that is present in almost all of our cells. DNA tells our cells (often indirectly) when to start growing, and when to stop; it defines the precise identity of each individual cell, forming anything from spindly electricity-conducting neurons to the armor-encased cells that shape our bones; and it creates the signaling molecules that shuttle between our cells to control their growth and architecture. This ancient molecule, which has persisted in some form for more than three billion years, carries the scars of its deep evolutionary history as well as our recent past—scientists can use DNA from an individual, for instance, to define almost exactly where their ancestors lived over the last few tens of thousands of years.

Despite this ancient pedigree, DNA remains vulnerable to particular changes. For most of the 20,000 or so genes found in the human genome, genetic changes that break those genes can have some effect on health or fitness. In many cases, particularly if a gene is completely broken in both copies (the one we inherit from our mother, and the second we inherit from our father) the result is severe disease. The impact of these genetic changes can vary enormously from gene to gene: changes in genes that help to protect muscle cells against damage can lead to muscular dystrophy; those in genes engaged in the formation of the infant brain, to developmental delay; those that control the growth and function of immune cells, to diseases that leave children vulnerable to infection by viruses, bacteria, or fungi. The links between specific genes and the rare diseases caused by losing them have taught us a great deal about human biology, even as they have inflicted suffering on millions of families.

The last five years have seen a resurgence of scientific interest in these disease. This has been driven in part by the development of remarkable new technologies for discovering the genetic causes of these diseases, which has dramatically transformed diagnosis rates for rare disease families, especially in those affected by the very rarest of diseases. Another driver has been a renewed interest from pharmaceutical companies in the development of therapies for rare diseases—an approach that was previously thought to be financially non-viable, but which has been opened up by changes in the U.S. regulatory framework and the economic model for drug development. Such changes have paved the way for genuinely transformative new therapies for a small number of rare diseases, including cystic fibrosis, spinal muscular atrophy, and degenerative eye diseases.

These scientific advances bring genuine hope—firstly that we will, over time, ultimately understand the biological basis of every rare genetic disease, and secondly that this understanding will ultimately lead us towards treatments for each and every such disease. But the road ahead remains hard. Despite our remarkable progress, more than half of the families affected by rare disease in the U.S. cannot be given a formal genetic diagnosis. More than half of the genes underlying these diseases remain unknown. And finally, and most importantly, the vast majority of all genetic diseases still have absolutely no effective therapy. Those of us in the scientific community are painfully aware of just how far we still need to go before we reach a world where no child suffers from genetic disease.

This remarkable book reminds us of exactly what we are fighting for. Every one of the tens of millions of rare disease patients around the world deserves a chance for a life free of fear and suffering. The faces in this book remind us of the bravery, and the hope, of rare disease families—and for those of us working on improving diagnosis or therapies, inspire us to work ever harder to change their lives.

Daniel MacArthur, PhD
Co-Director, Medical and Population Genetics, Broad Institute of MIT and Harvard
Assistant Professor, Harvard Medical School and Massachusetts General Hospital

Introduction

One of my earliest memories as a little girl is going through my mother's drawer and finding photographs of a baby that wasn't me or my brother. When I asked her who it was, she told me about Rafi. Rafi was my mother's firstborn, and he died of Tay-Sachs disease before reaching the age of three.

As immigrants, my parents didn't have many people or places to turn to when my brother was diagnosed, so they went to a Tay-Sachs support group. My mother later spent years as the president of the Queens, New York chapter, running raffles, bazaars, and galas to raise money and awareness. While there is still no cure for Tay-Sachs, there is now far more information available to families at risk. Today, Jewish parents are screened for the Tay-Sachs gene during pregnancy, decreasing the occurrence.

It wasn't until years later, when I became a mother, that I could really understand my mother's pain. Losing a child contradicts the cycle of life. Children are supposed to outlive their parents. Any other sequence of events is simply unbearable. Almost fifty years later, my parents still suffer from the loss of their son Rafi.

More recently, my best friend's son Ethan was diagnosed with Angelman syndrome—a rare disease that primarily affects the nervous system. While Ethan's syndrome is not terminal, he requires constant care. Hearing of the hardship her family is forced to confront daily made me realize a spotlight needs to be put on families like these. Though each family struggles alone, countless families confront similar anguish, difficulty, and abiding love. And so my project began.

Rare genetic diseases are more common than the label implies. According to Global Genes, one out of ten Americans is affected, while 95% of rare diseases do not have an FDA-approved drug treatment. But rare genetic diseases impact more than just those diagnosed: parents, siblings, friends, and extended family members all feel their worlds shake.

At the onset of my project, I asked several organizations working with these families if they would help me spread the word. I wondered if parents and children would be willing to share their stories and let me and my camera into their homes for a day. The positive response was tremendous.

The families that are in this book all want to educate the world about their children's diseases. They want to raise awareness in any way they can—and this book is an outlet. Through these photographs, I hope to give a voice to families raising children with rare genetic disorders and capture their lives in all their simplicity and humanity. I aim to raise awareness, tolerance, and support for these children and their loved ones.

Each family is on their own journey with their own set of symptoms, yet, they have a lot in common. They all faced that moment when they realized that their children are not typical. While many do not ever get a proper diagnosis, those who do remember that moment often referred to it as "D Day" (Diagnosis Day)—when many of their hopes and dreams for their child were shattered and they shifted into a new reality.

All of the families interviewed are fighting for the best care for their children. Many are battling insurance companies for services at home to help their children develop the skills they need to survive. They exude resilience, hope, and patience. Each day there are struggles and victories, joys and sorrows. As Stephanie says about her son, "We are just working toward making Ethan the best Ethan he can be."

There are many unanswerable questions in the world of rare diseases. The families I met live with excruciating uncertainties every day of their lives. *Will my child be able to walk, talk, and be potty trained? Will he or she have a social life or a job? Who will take care of them when I am not around?* Or, even more unfathomable,*Will I outlive them?*

Aside from the medical struggles, I've found that families touched by rare illnesses often battle a sense of isolation from their communities. Society doesn't deal well with "different." Many of the children experience bullying, staring, and being shunned. A moment of uncontrolled bodily movement or an unprompted loud noise frequently leads adults and kids to step away or look with judgment, rather than lean in and ask a question, or smile. The intimate portraits in *An Ordinary Day* inspire hope, empathy, and appreciation in all of us.

The chronic illness of a child requires a family's total commitment every moment of every day. It requires time to battle insurance companies, search for support, and very often, struggle with everyday tasks that others perform effortlessly. But coping can also provide moments of profound dignity, grace, and joy. *An Ordinary Day* provides a record of such moments, illuminating what it means to be a family, as well as what it means to be human, regardless of health or lifespan.

Collaborating with these families has been a life-changing gift for me. They have given me perspective, taught me what real patience looks like, forced me to reconsider what it means to parent, and inspired me to reevaluate what is important in this life. I am humbled by their resilience, how strong and courageous these children are, and how much fight they bring to each day's challenges—often without tears and, instead, with a smile on their face. It has been a privilege to enter each family's world, hear their stories, and meet their beautiful children. This book is dedicated to them.

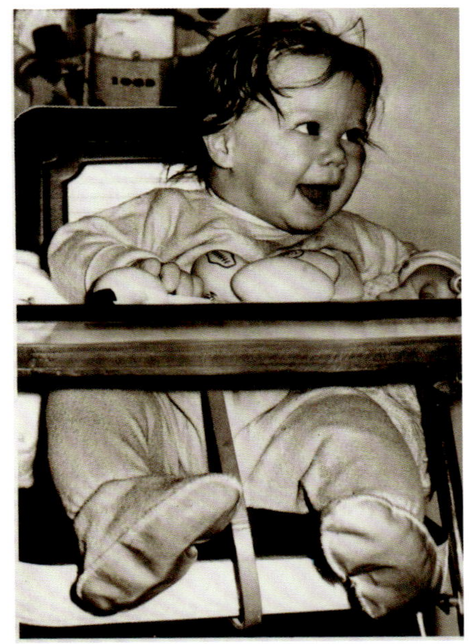

RAPHAEL HABERBERG — 5/13/66 - 5/10/69

WYATT LOVES TO STARE AT SMALL THINGS LIKE STICKS.

Wyatt

Wyatt, 5, is missing a piece of his 22nd chromosome—a mutation that can manifest itself in many ways. Wyatt is nonverbal, cannot eat by mouth, and is blind in one eye. Two of his fingers are fused together on one hand. He has already had eight surgeries, including one open-heart surgery. Wyatt loves the outdoors. He is very tactile and enjoys nature, the pool, and obstacle courses.

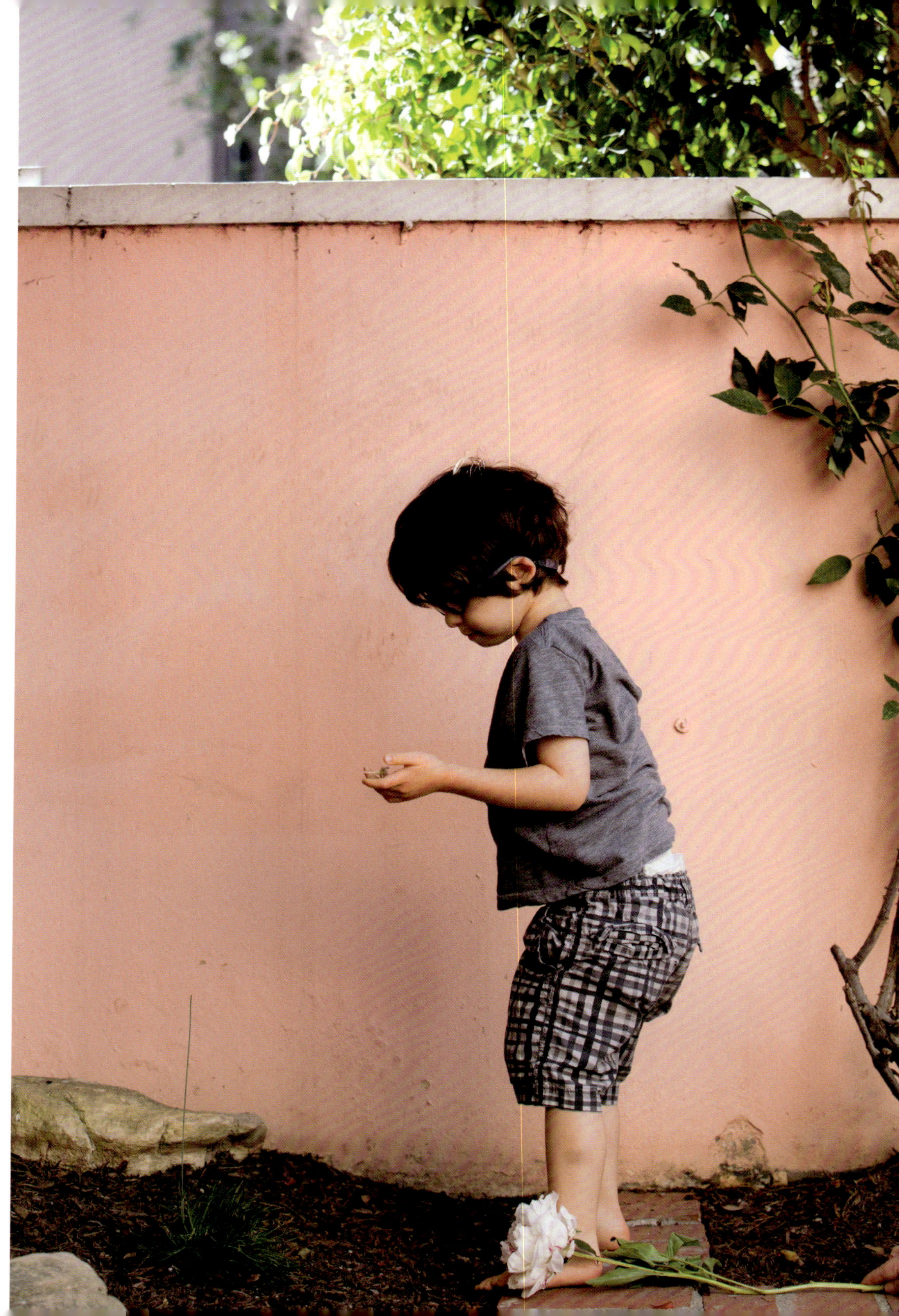

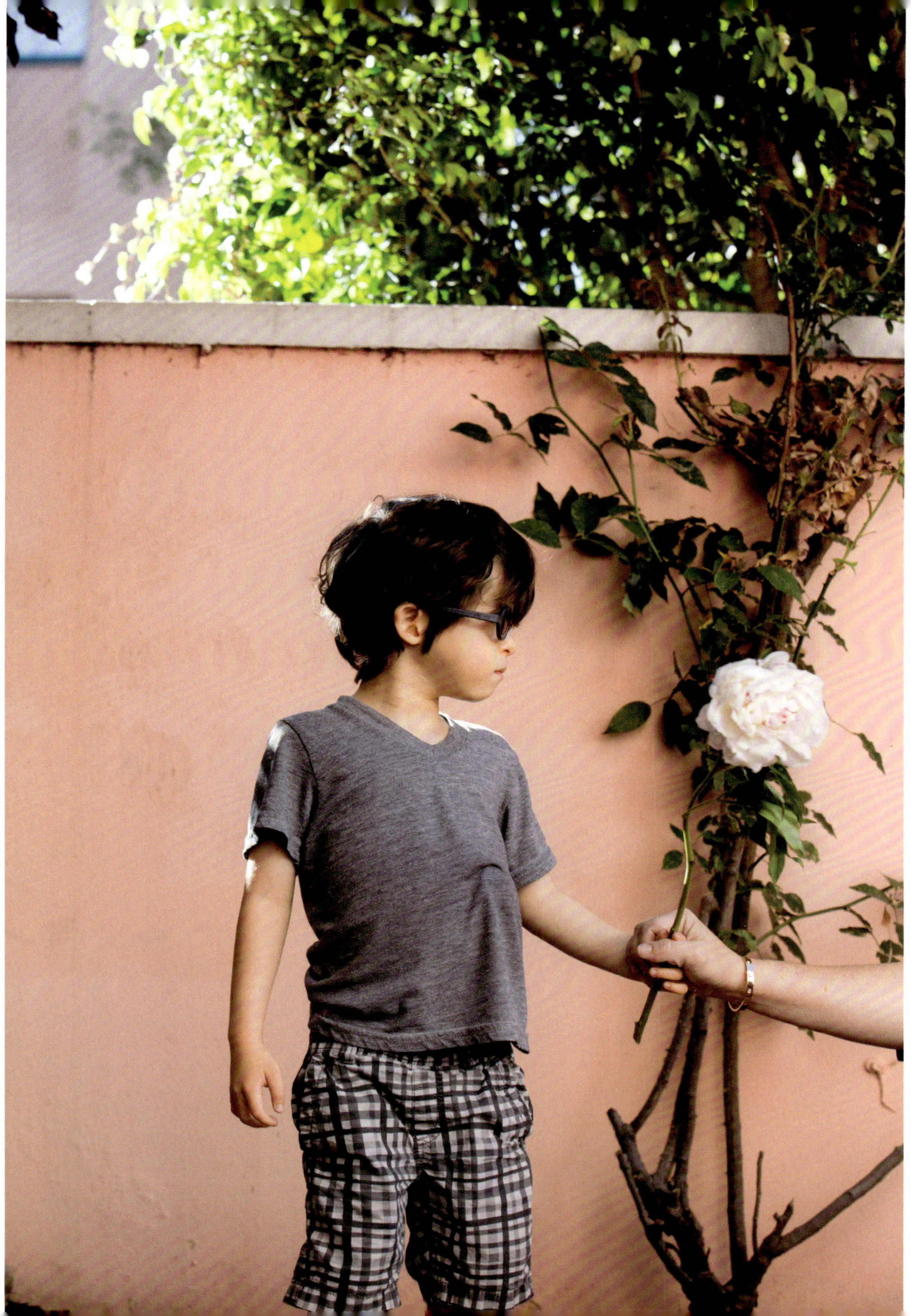

Obviously we were crushed but we didn't even realize then what it meant for a while. The hospital that he was born at didn't really know what it meant, so we didn't really know what it meant. And then as it went on we kept learning more and more. – Sally, Wyatt's mother

*They had a Wikipedia printout of his syndrome, that was their guidance for treating him in the first place.
– Brian, Wyatt's father*

I remember when I said to my friend, "Wyatt learned to put objects in a bucket today," and she was like, "I didn't even know that was a thing, my kid just did it. I didn't realize it was like a thing to learn." So for me it's so great to recognize every little step as being fantastic and being so excited about things that other people wouldn't notice. – Sally, Wyatt's mother

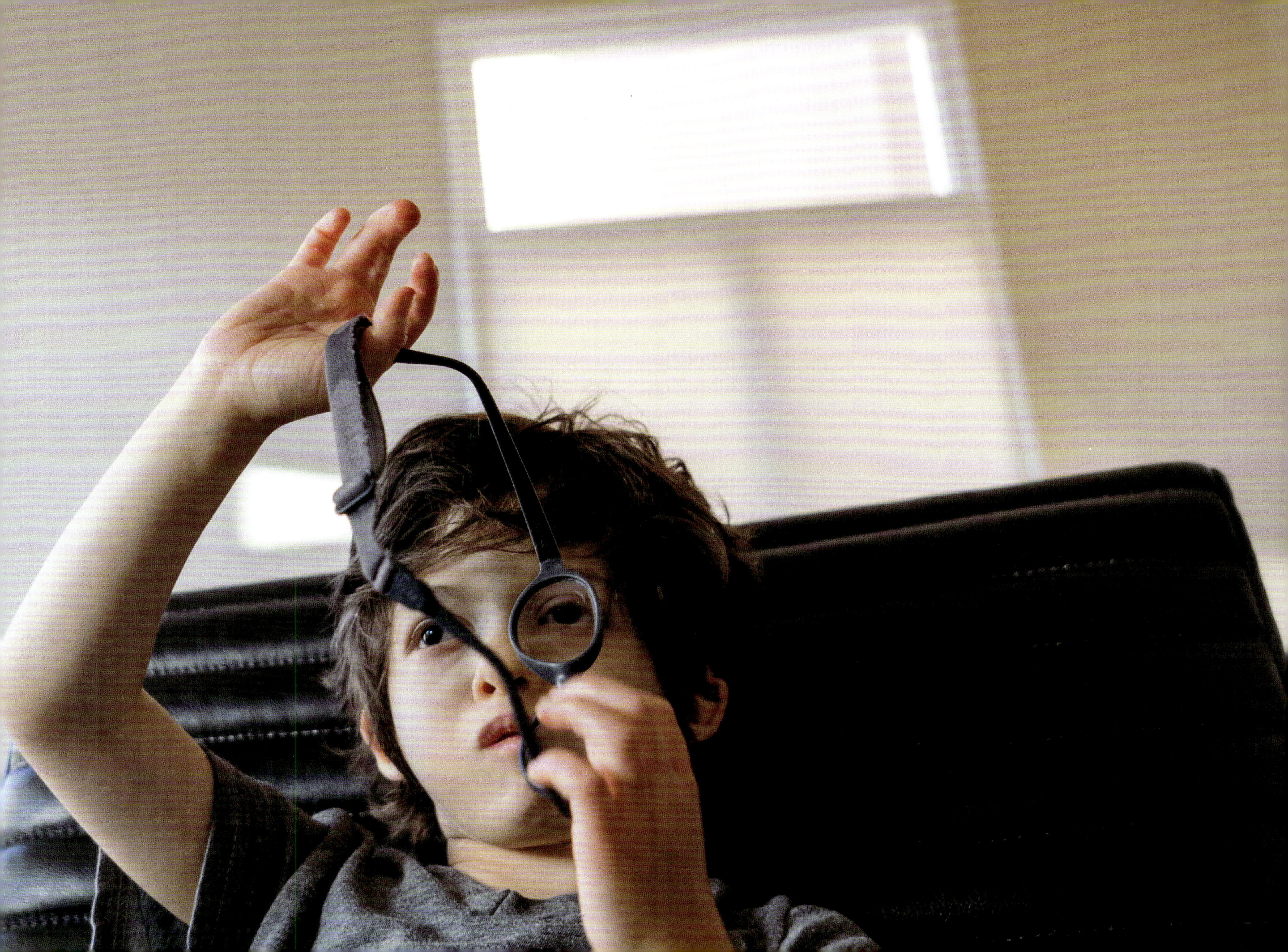

Cassie

The first time Cassie's parents heard the words Marfan syndrome, their daughter was about five hours old. Marfan syndrome is a genetic disorder that affects the body's connective tissue, causing features such as long limbs, a curved spine, a tall and thin body type, and a dilated aortic root, which can be fatal if not diagnosed in time. Cassie, 9, has had six surgeries, including heart surgery, three spinal surgeries, g-tube placement, and a fix of her broken femur. Due to the metal rods along her spine, which correct her scoliosis, she cannot bend her back. Cassie loves to sing and act, swim, and play Minecraft.

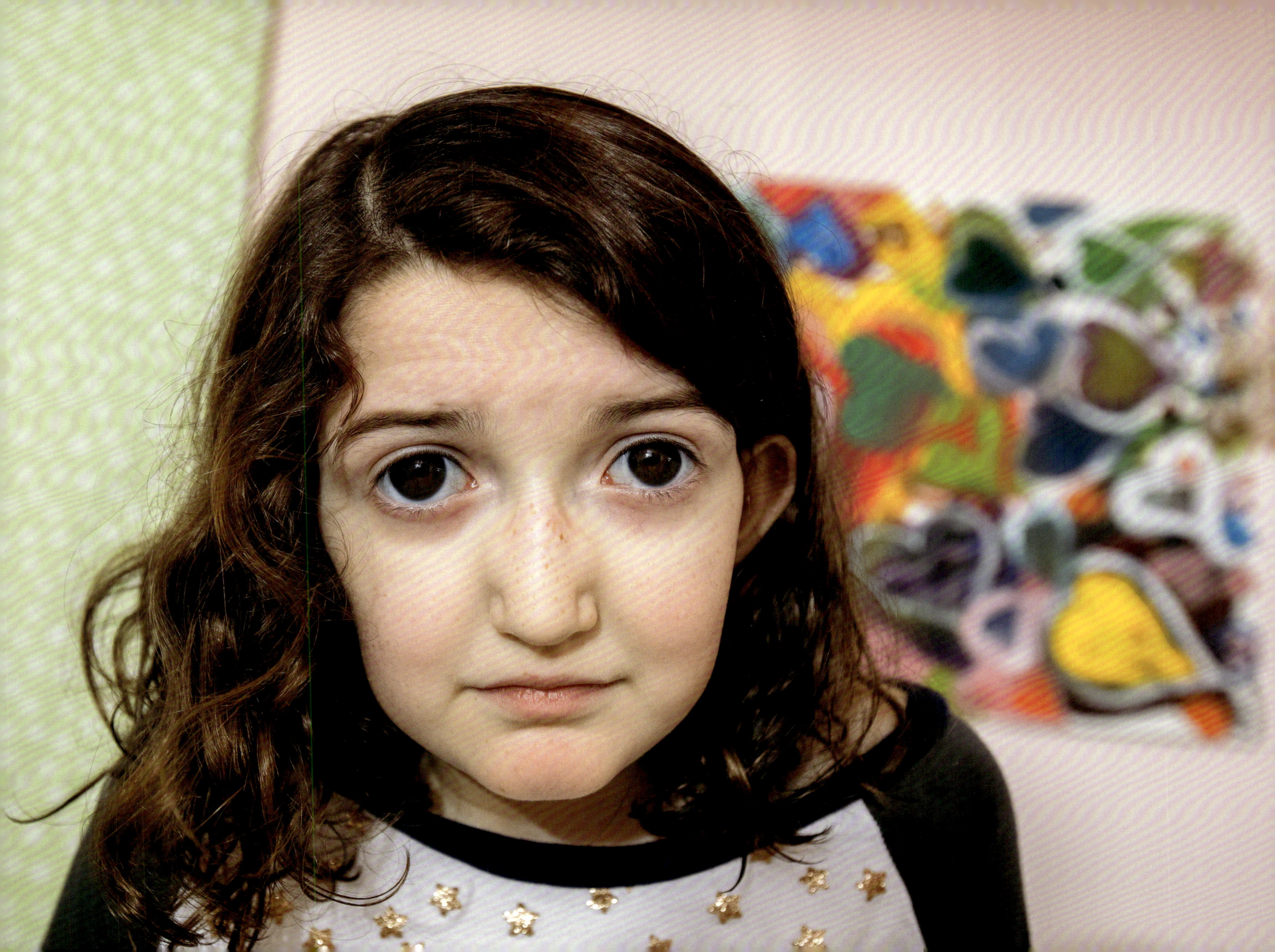

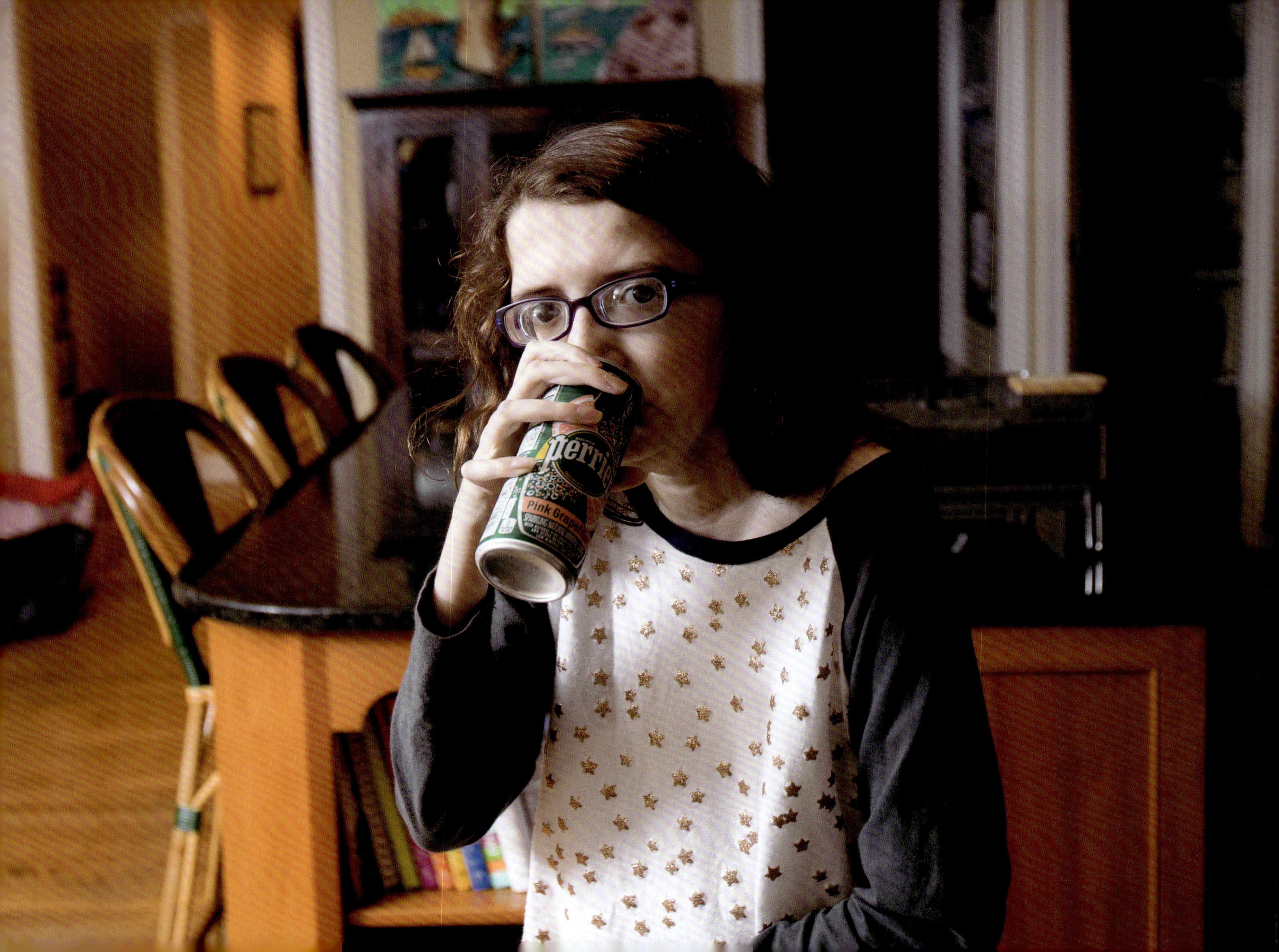
perrier

For Cassie in the day to day, there are tough things with friends at school. She can't do what they can do on the playground. She wants to run around and she can't keep up, which is tough. Her friends are sweet to her, but they're also nine-year-olds who want to run around at recess. That's a very tough thing to figure out. –Alix, Cassie's mother

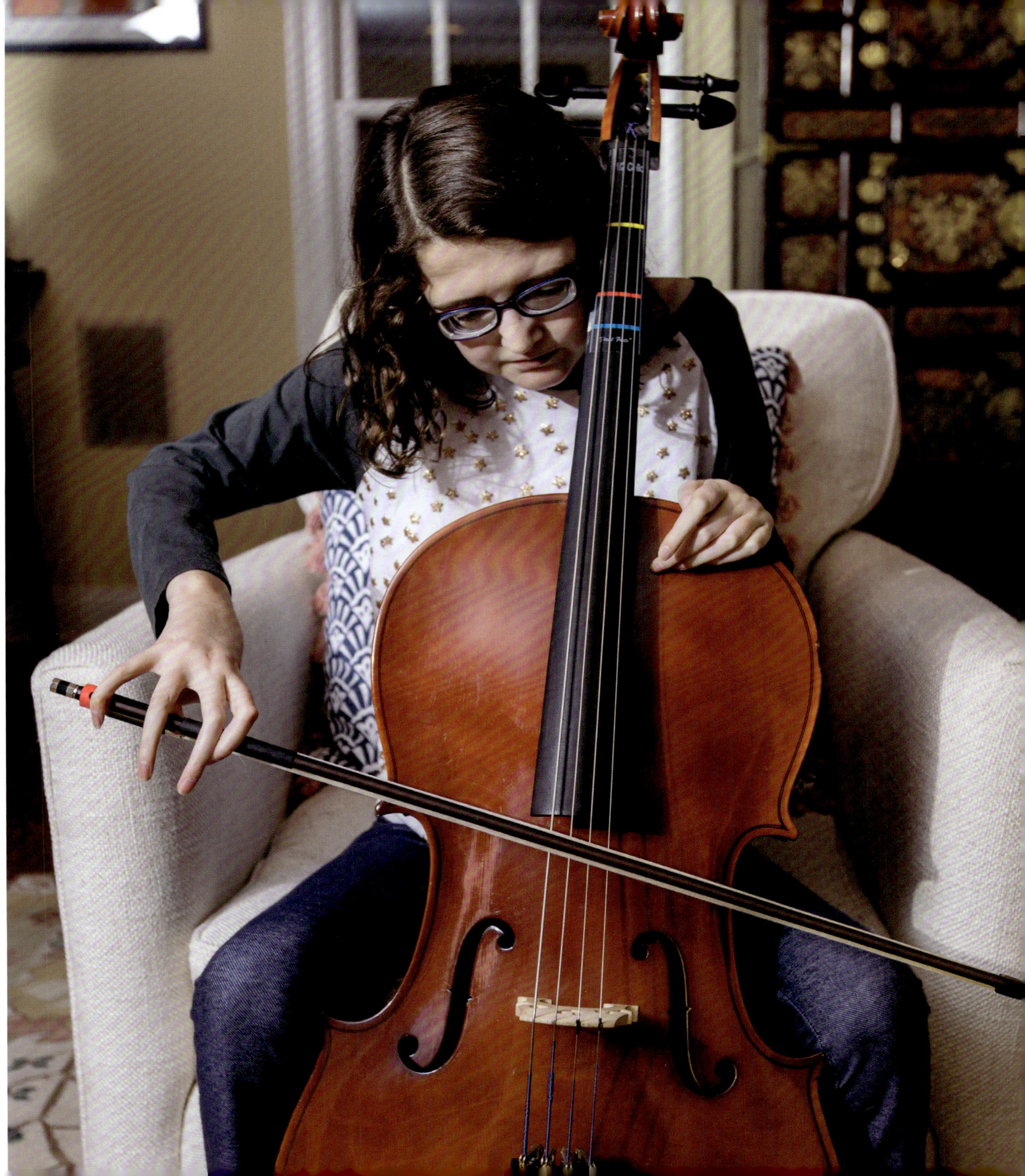

If she drops her pencil on the floor, she has trouble getting it because she can't bend her back. Some kids are really great about grabbing things for her and helping her out. She doesn't even have to ask them, they just do it. One boy, Matthew, protects her during gym sometimes, diving in front of balls he thinks might hit her. –Alix, Cassie's mother

One time last year on the playground when I was in line to go on the swings, there was a girl that asked me why I was so tall. I either said, "I don't want to talk about it," "It's complicated," or "I was born this way." She must have had some clue about the surgeries and stuff because she said, "Why, because you've had like a hundred surgeries or something?" That made me really mad.
– Cassie

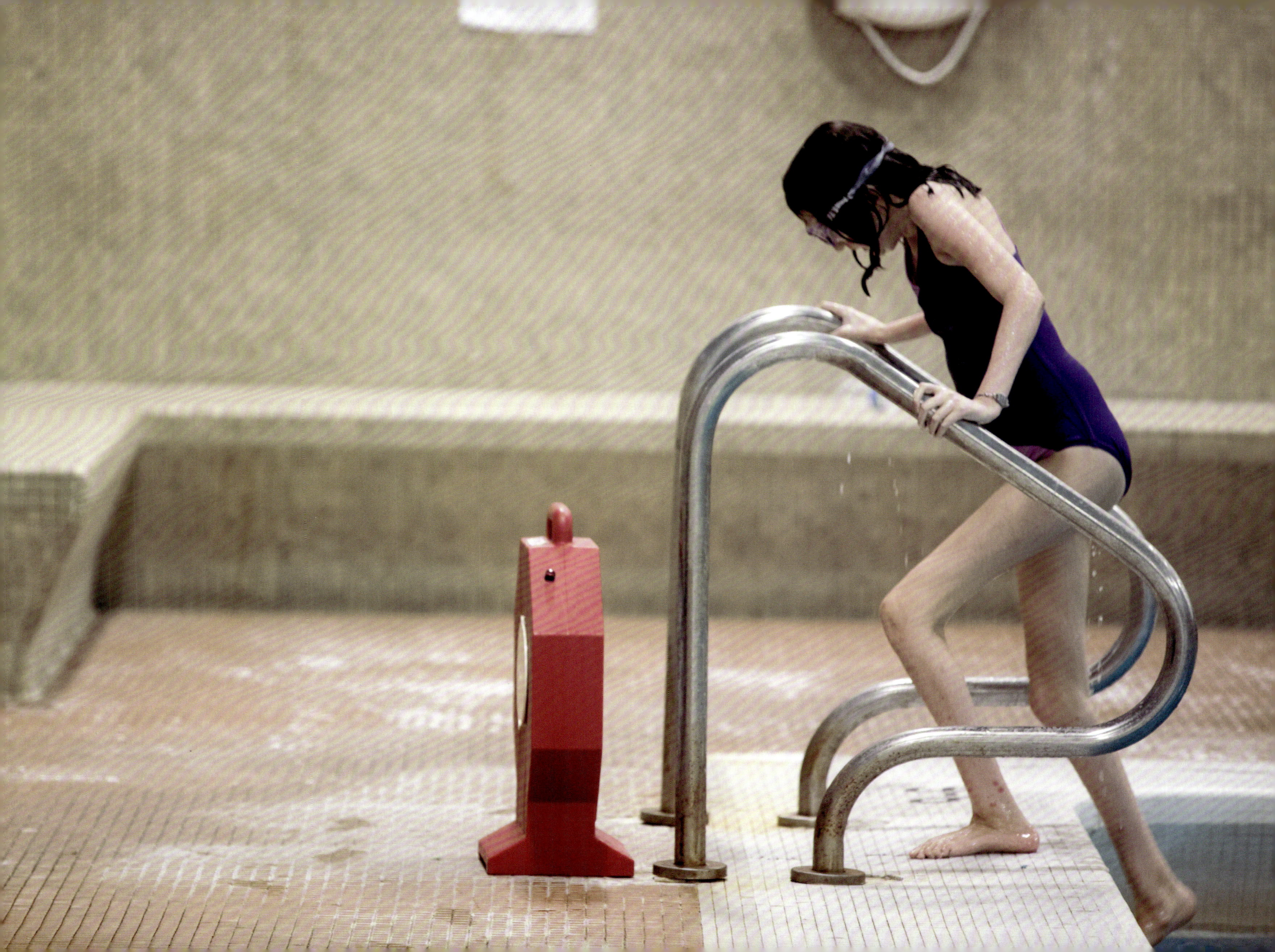

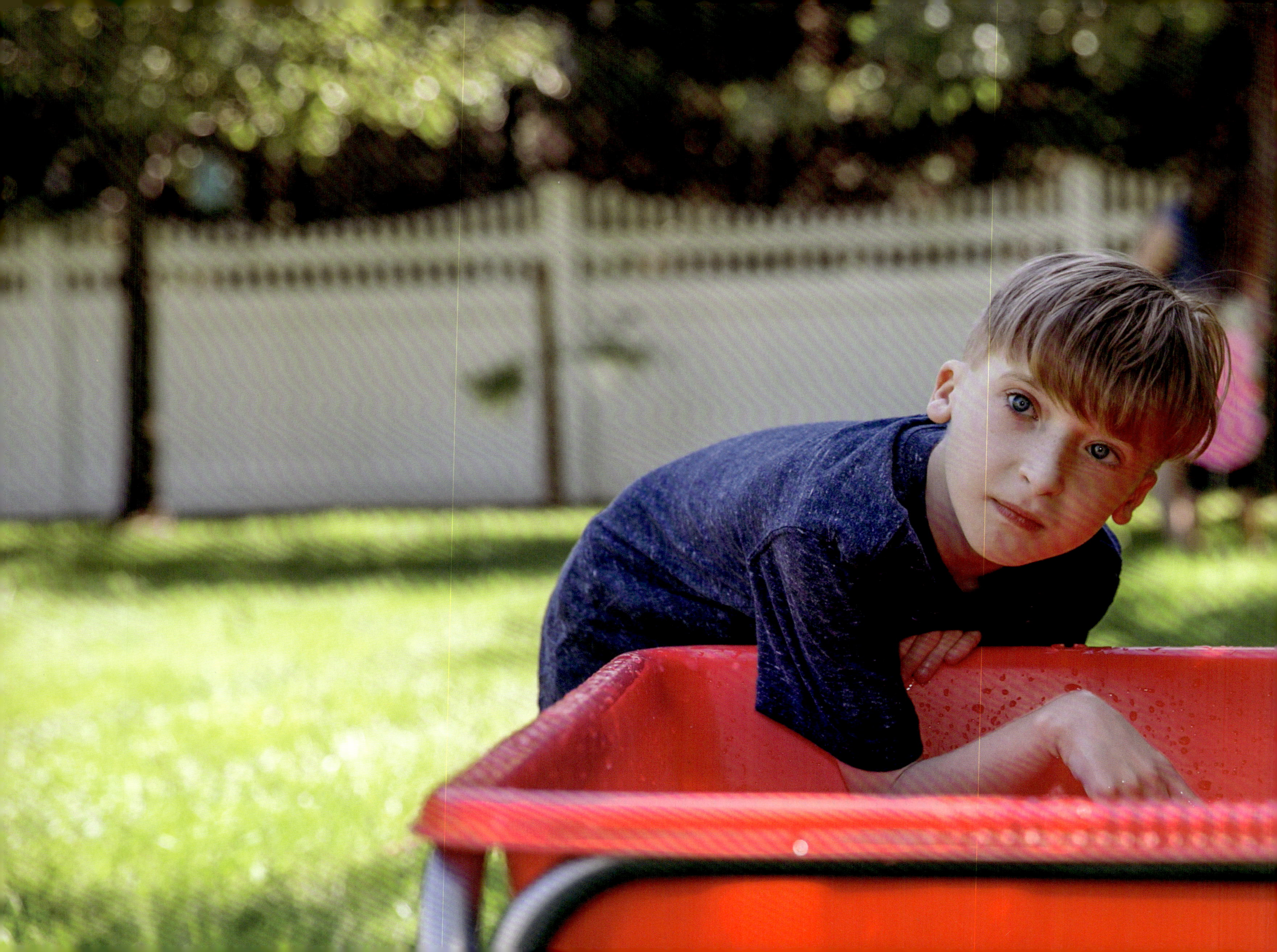

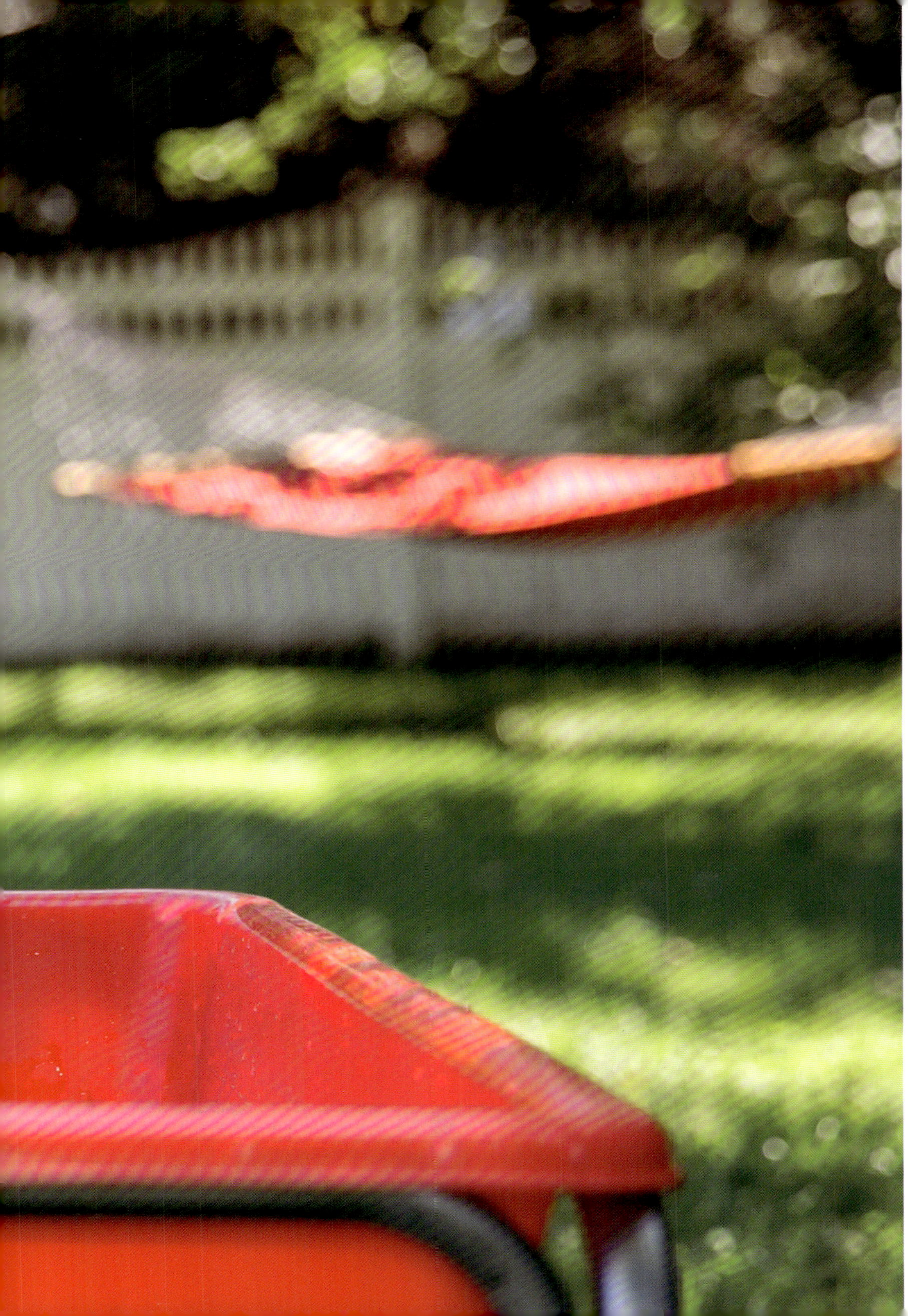

Jonathan

Jonathan, 9, has Mowat-Wilson syndrome, an incredibly rare condition that was discovered in 1998. As a result of his condition, Jonathan cannot talk. Though he is capable of eating soft foods, he generally does not like to eat and is not able to self-feed. He also recently began having seizures. Jonathan loves watching football and listening to live music.

Because it's so rare, there's no real documentation. There were no other cases that we could look at. In the beginning, we did find a few families here and there, but that was it. We kind of had to do what we felt was right and what he was responding to and take it day by day. – Jessica, Jonathan's mother

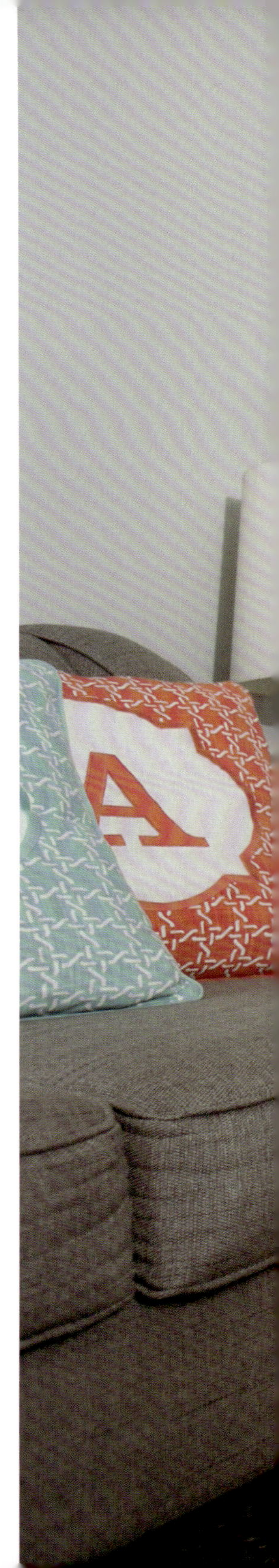

JONATHAN LOVES TO WATCH LIVE AND RECORDED NEW YORK JETS' GAMES.

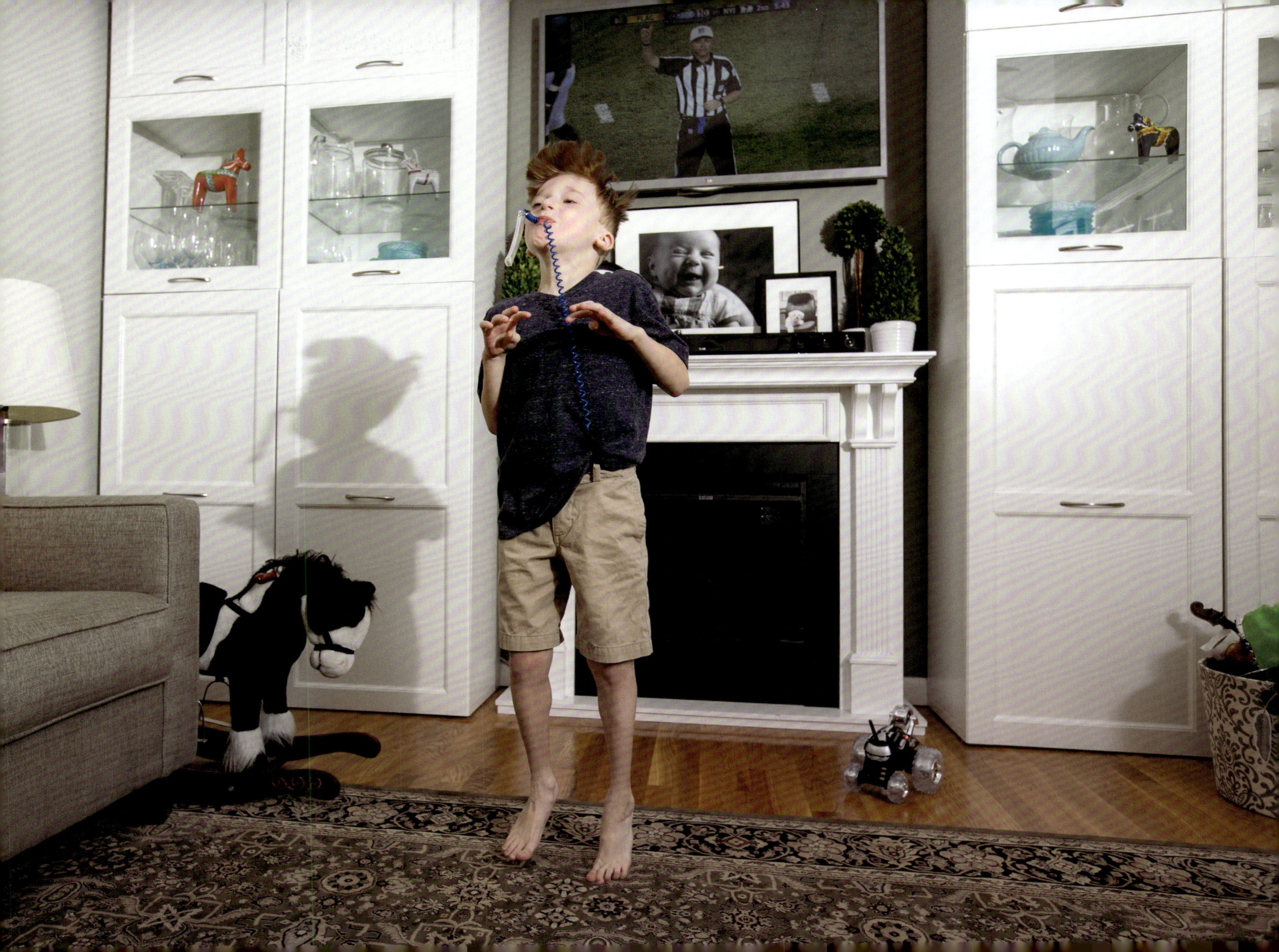

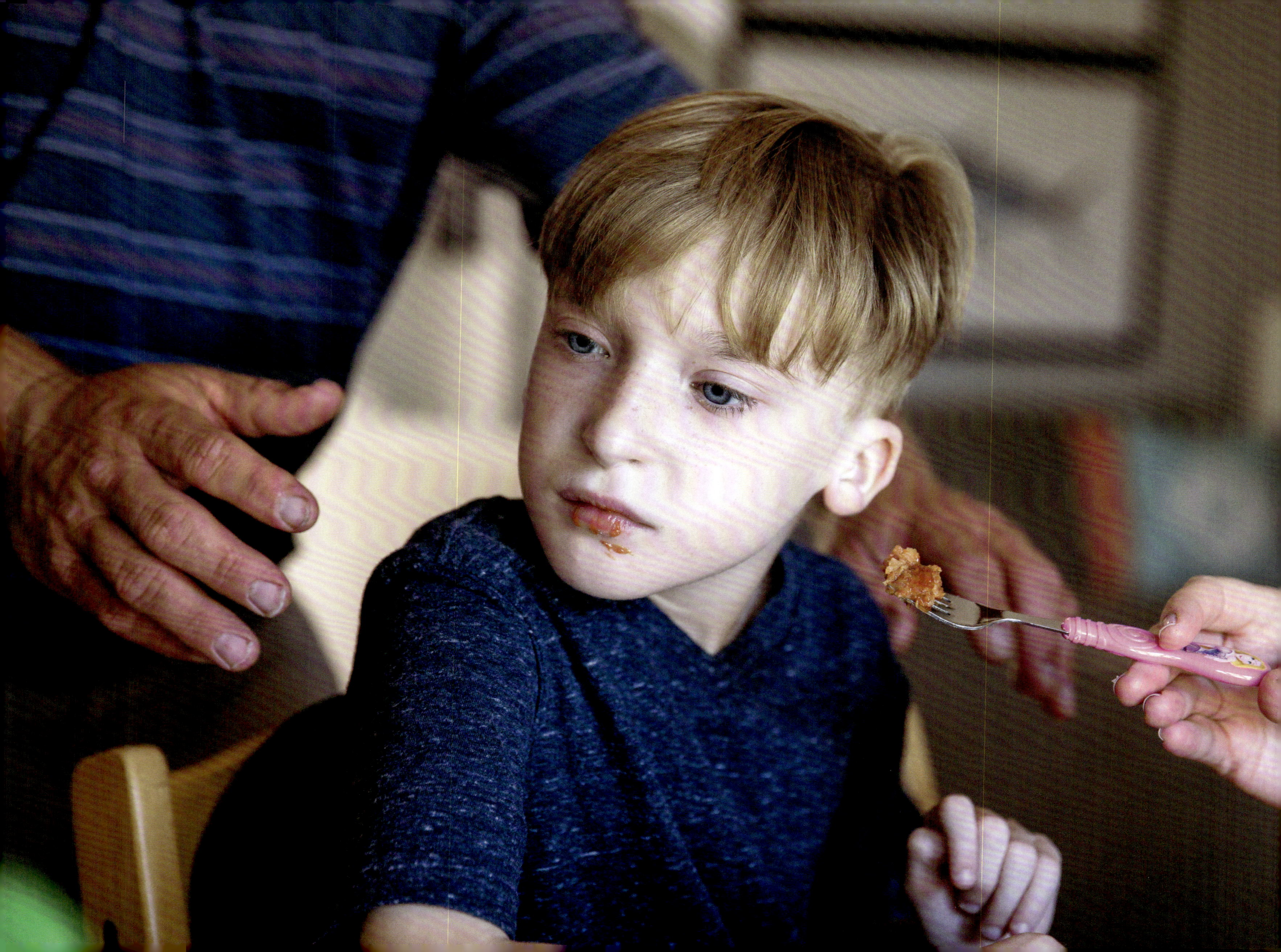

He doesn't like to eat. He can probably eat anything. He can swallow and chew. He has a high tolerance for pain. When we get a little bit hungry, we want to feed that pain. When he gets hungry, it's a massive issue because he hasn't eaten in a very long time. Then he doesn't know how to control it. – Jessica, Jonathan's mom

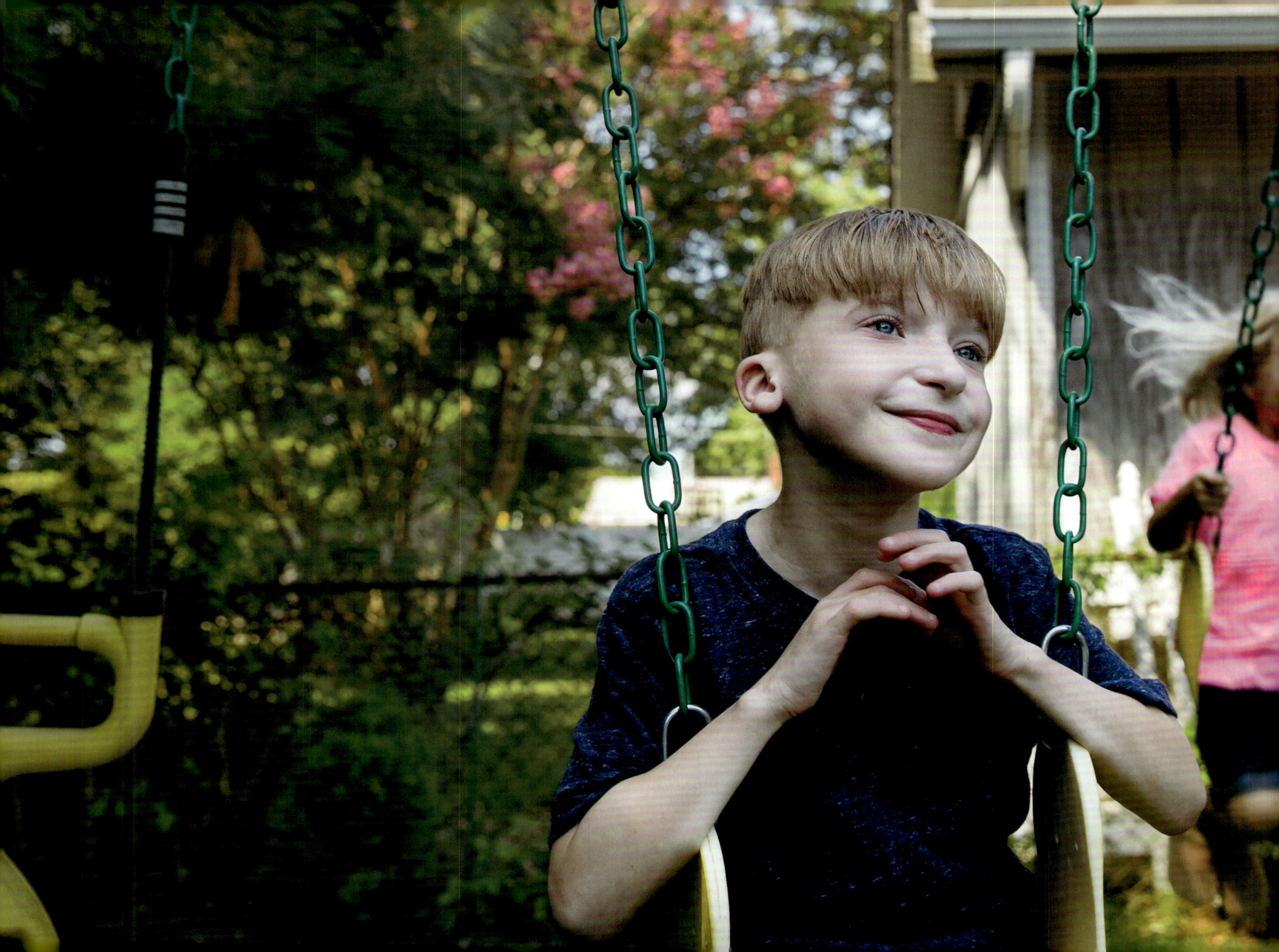

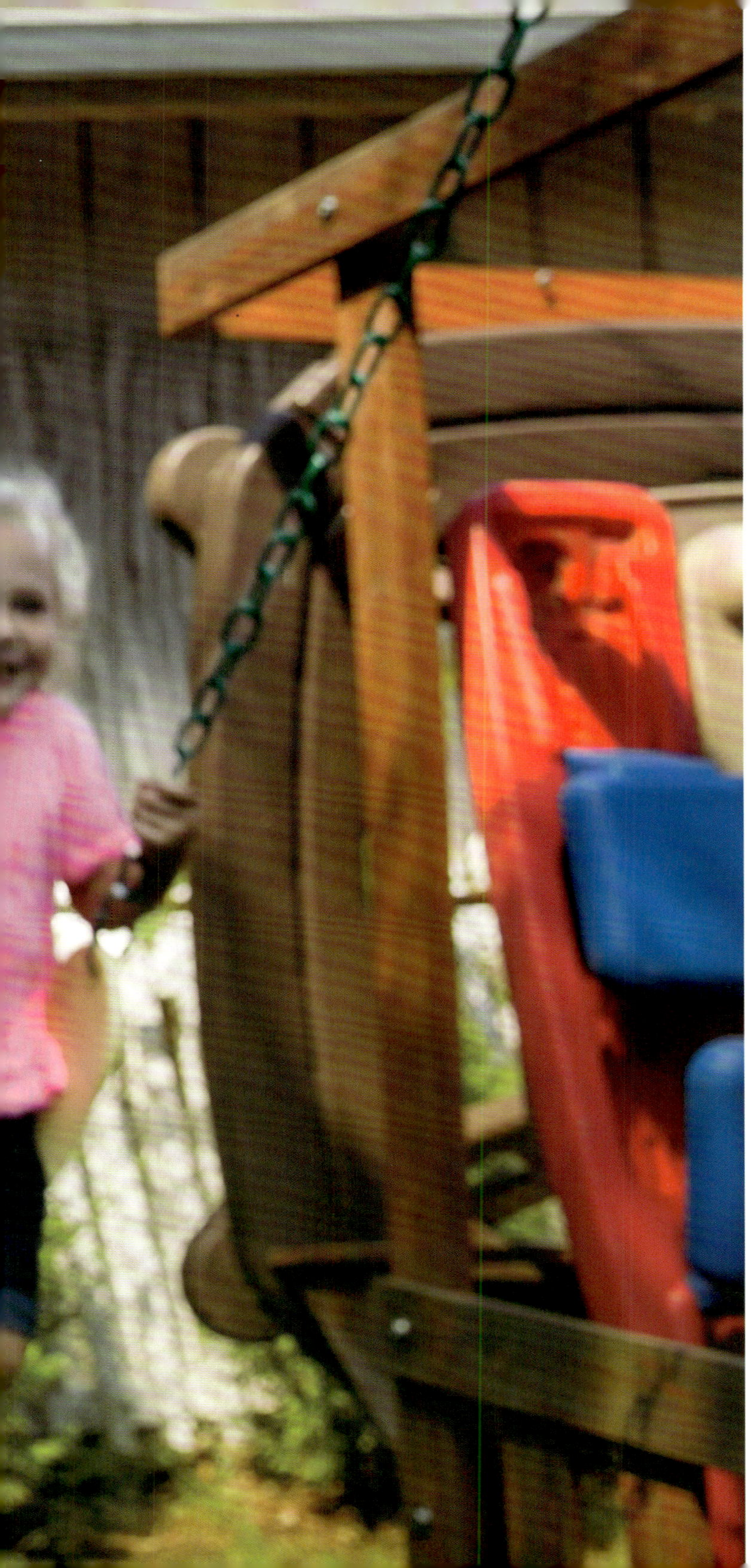

[Jonathan's sister] had never really known that he wasn't talking to her this whole time because they communicate in their own way. She never actually thought about it. It was like it blew her mind. Steam was coming out. She was four and a half years old when I told her. Now, she's starting to realize that she's helping me with him in the bathtub and cleaning his room and making him smile and all sorts of stuff. I think she still has a bit to learn. She's only five but she's starting to know it's different and it's okay. It's how we are.
– Jessica, Jonathan's mom

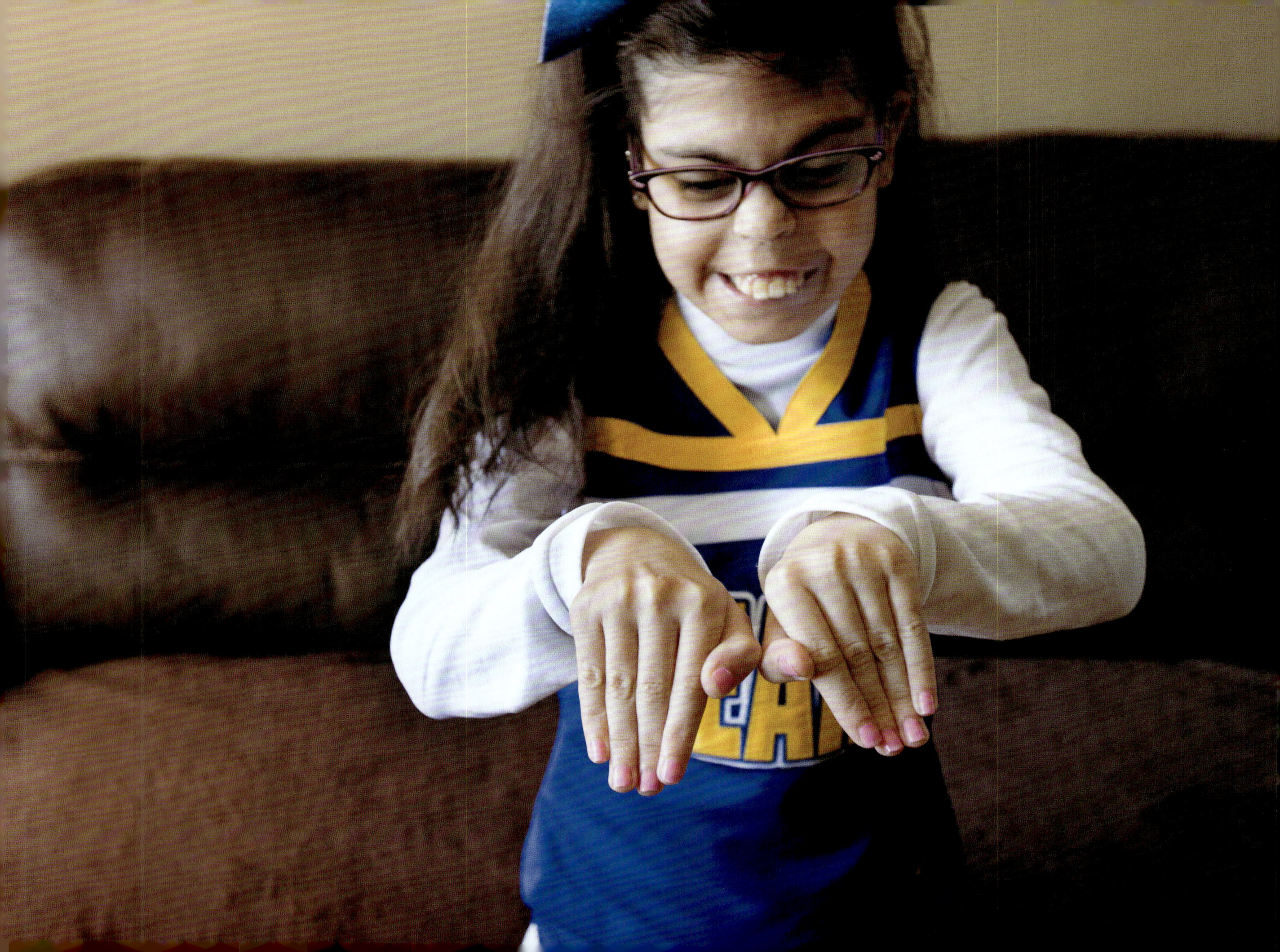

I asked Gianna what she likes about cheering. She said, "I love the uniform and hanging out with girls and doing stunts. I like to be with friends." As her mom I think what strikes me most is her saying, "to be with friends." She doesn't have "friends" in the regular sense of the word. She doesn't do playdates or sleepovers or go hang out like the typical girls her age. So when she goes to cheer she is around other girls, so to her, that's being "with friends."
– Anna, Gianna's mother

Gianna

At just 20 weeks, while in utero, Gianna was diagnosed with 22q11.2 deletion syndrome. At just three days old she had nasal surgery, and then at two months old, heart surgery. To date, she has had 26 surgeries. Gianna, 14, suffers from seizures, feeding and swallowing issues, growth deficiency, bowel and bladder incontinence, cognitive delays, OCD, ADD, and Tourettes spectrum, among many other things. Despite this, Gianna is always enthusiastic; her favorite activity is cheering.

Gianna takes things very literally. Last year leading up to her 13th birthday everyone was making a big deal that now she is a teenager and so grown up. She came to me at the end of the day on her birthday teary eyed and said, "Mommy, I looked in the mirror and I thought, how come I don't look like the girls in my class? I didn't get boobies. I thought I was going to look older and bigger like the girls in my class." She had thought that she would miraculously look like the girls who are her age. It broke my heart. – Anna, Gianna mother

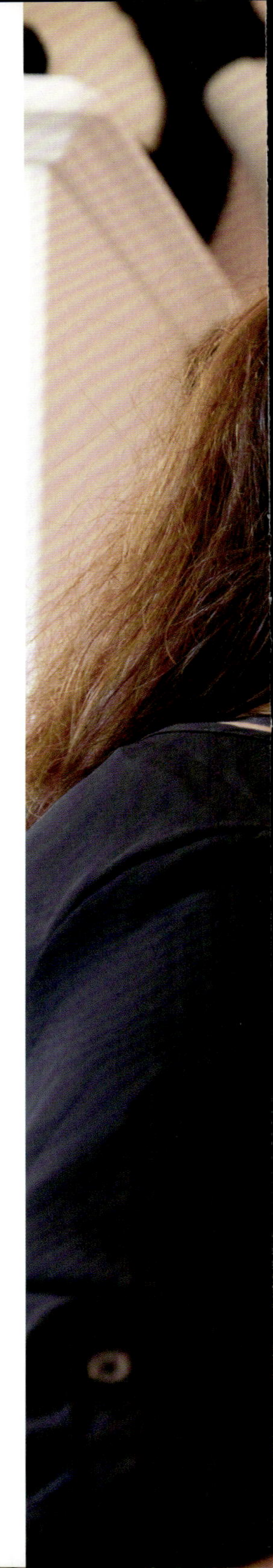

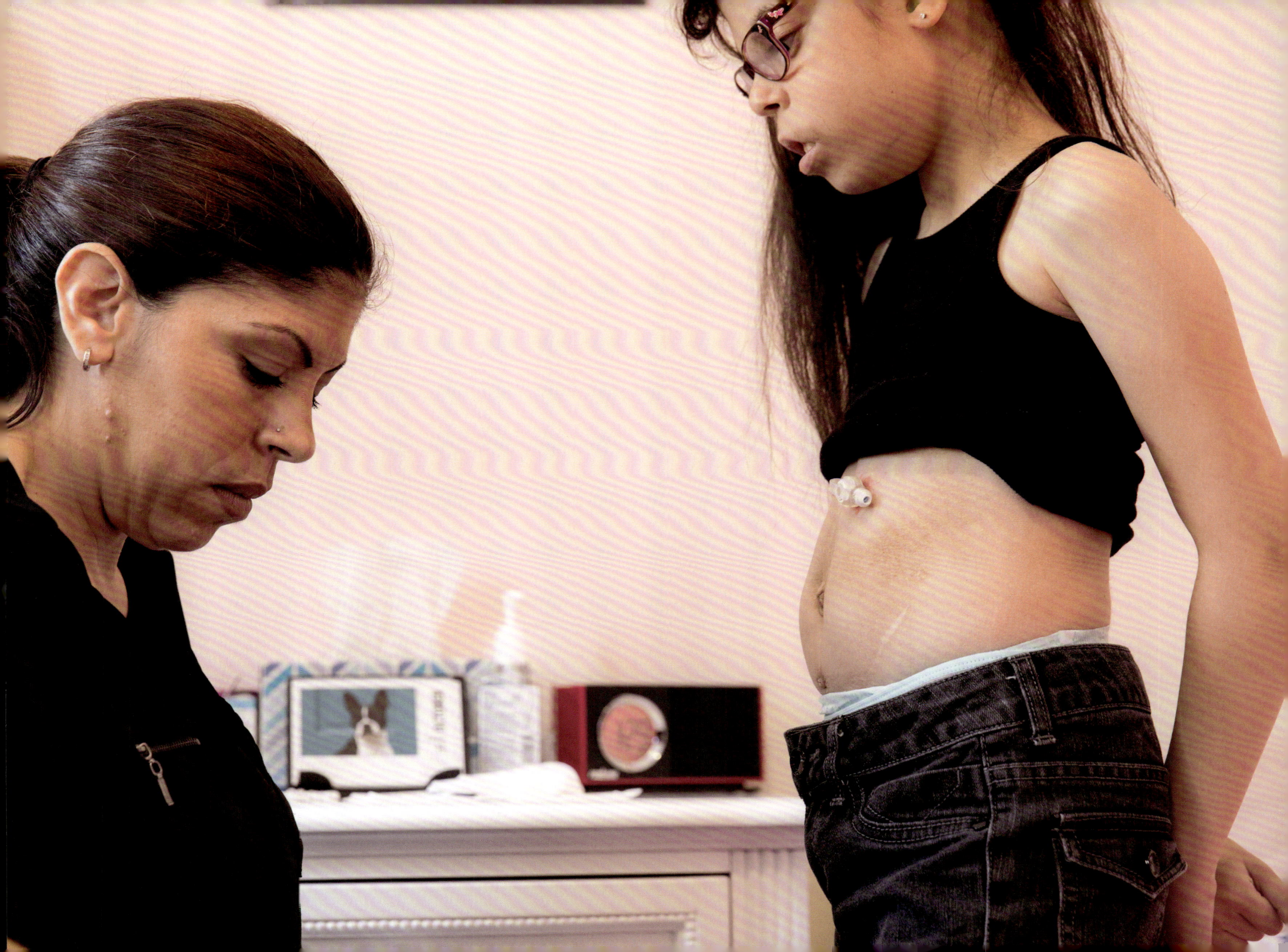

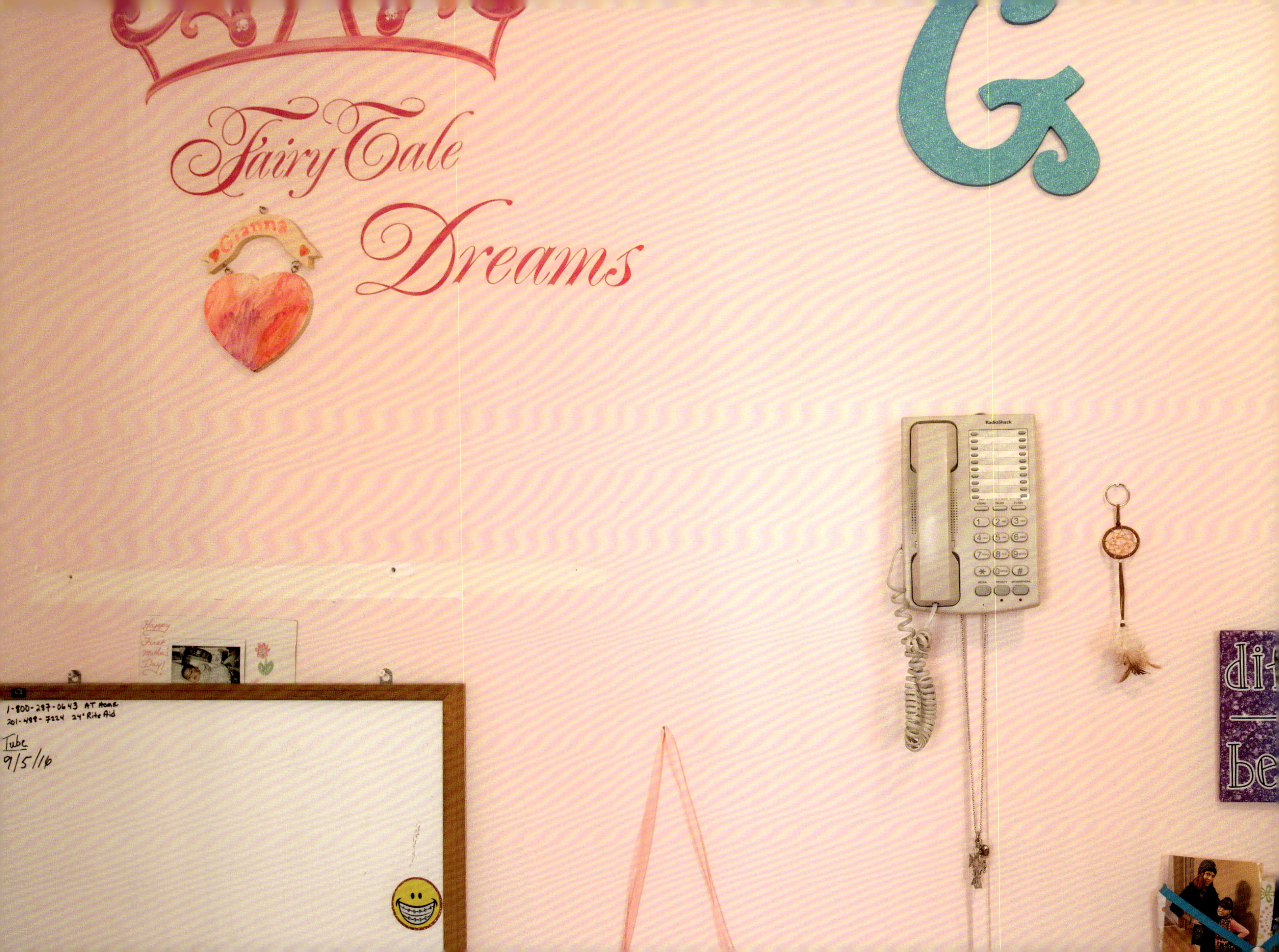
Fairy Tale
Dreams
Gianna
G
RadioShack
Happy First Mother's Day!
1-800-287-0643 AT Home
201-488-7224 24° Rite Aid
Tube
9/5/16

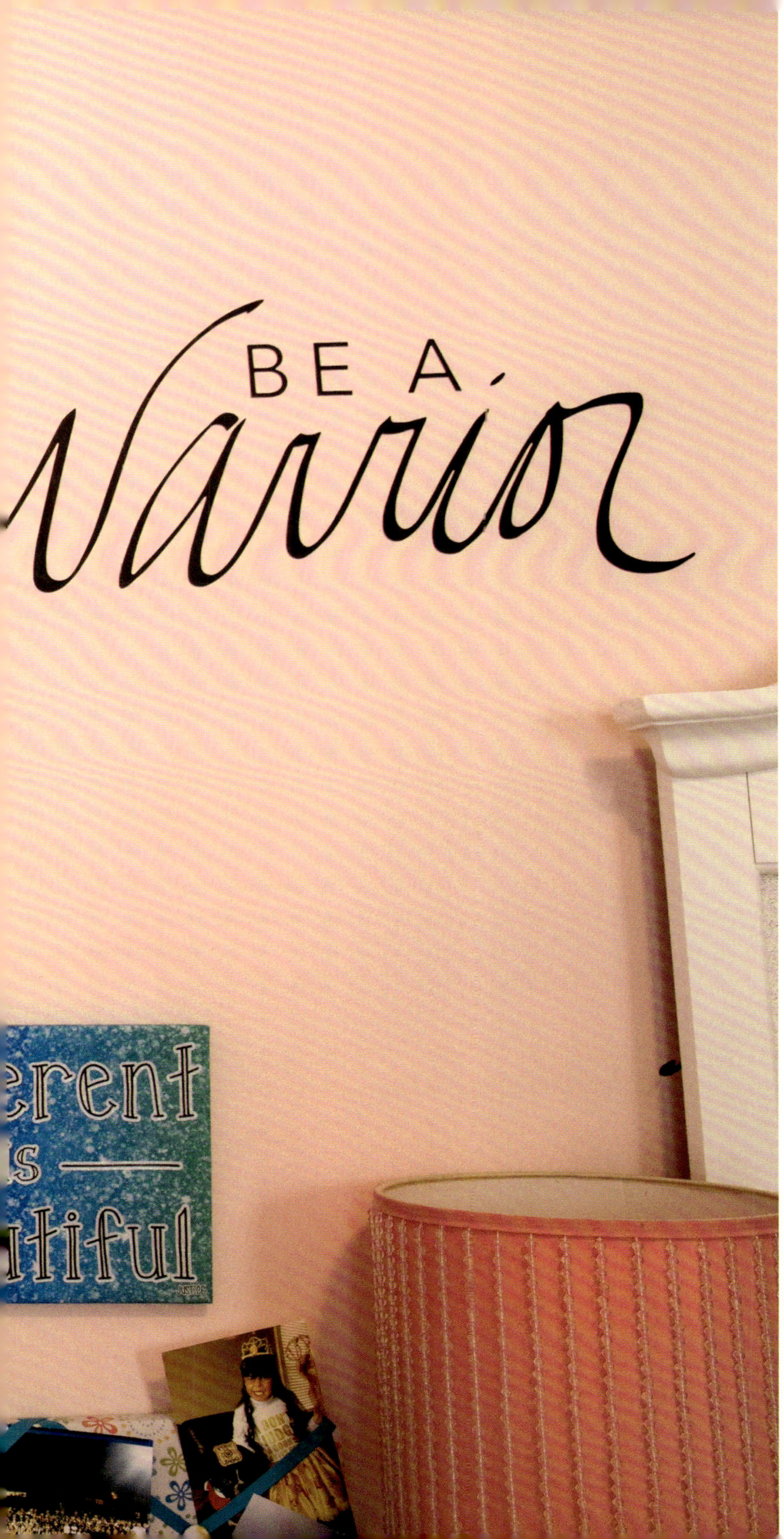

She is my shining example of life, inspiration, and gratitude. In this lifetime she will be able to teach me more than I will ever be able to teach her.
– Anna, Gianna's mother

Our mission as Team G [Gianna's tightknit circle of family and friends] is to educate all about tolerance, acceptance, and inclusion. We tell Gianna all the time, and she repeats back to us, 'Different is beautiful!'
– Anna, Gianna's mother

IN GIANNA'S ROOM, A LAND-LINE PHONE WAS INSTALLED FOR MEDICAL EMERGENCIES.

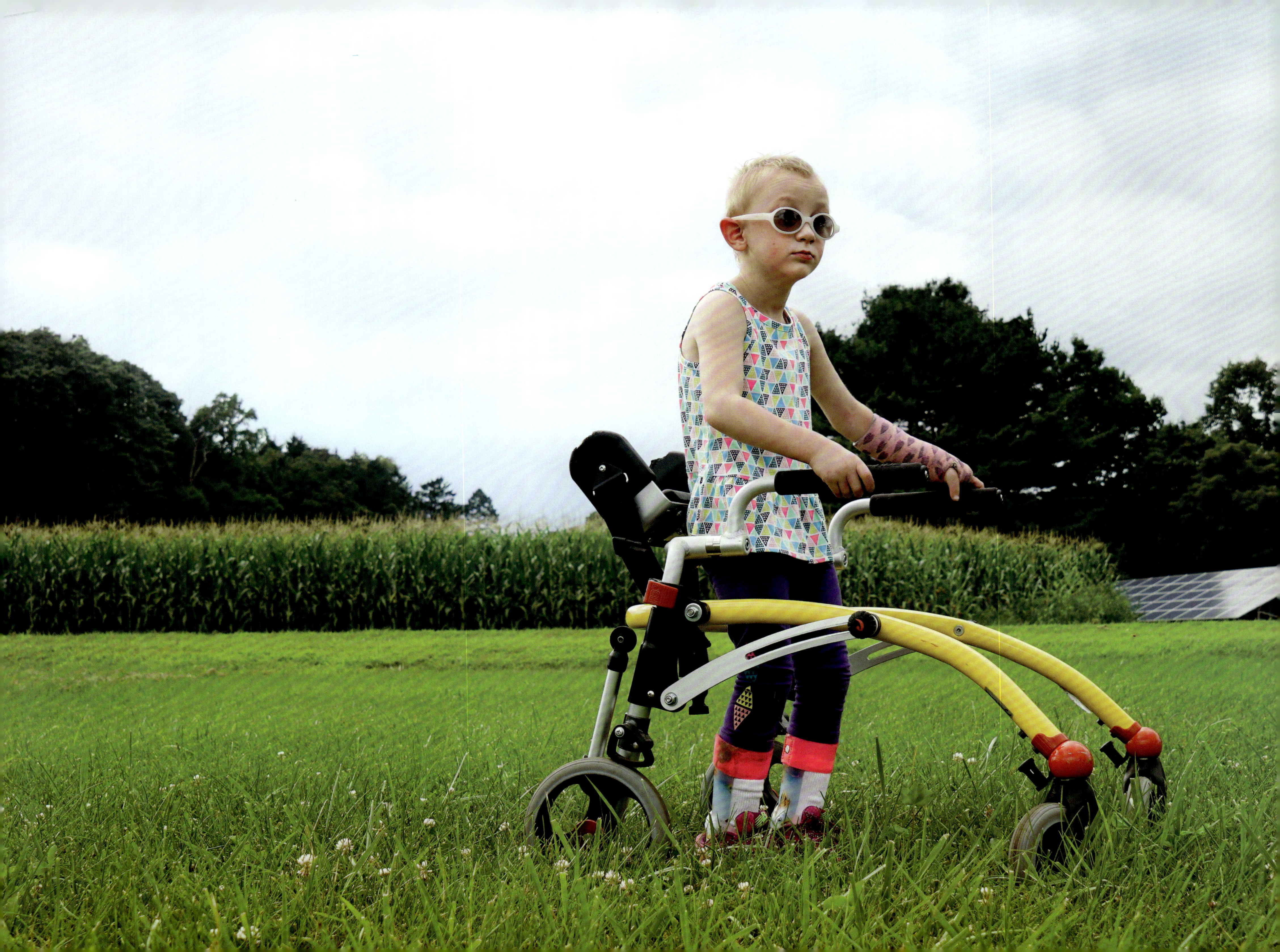

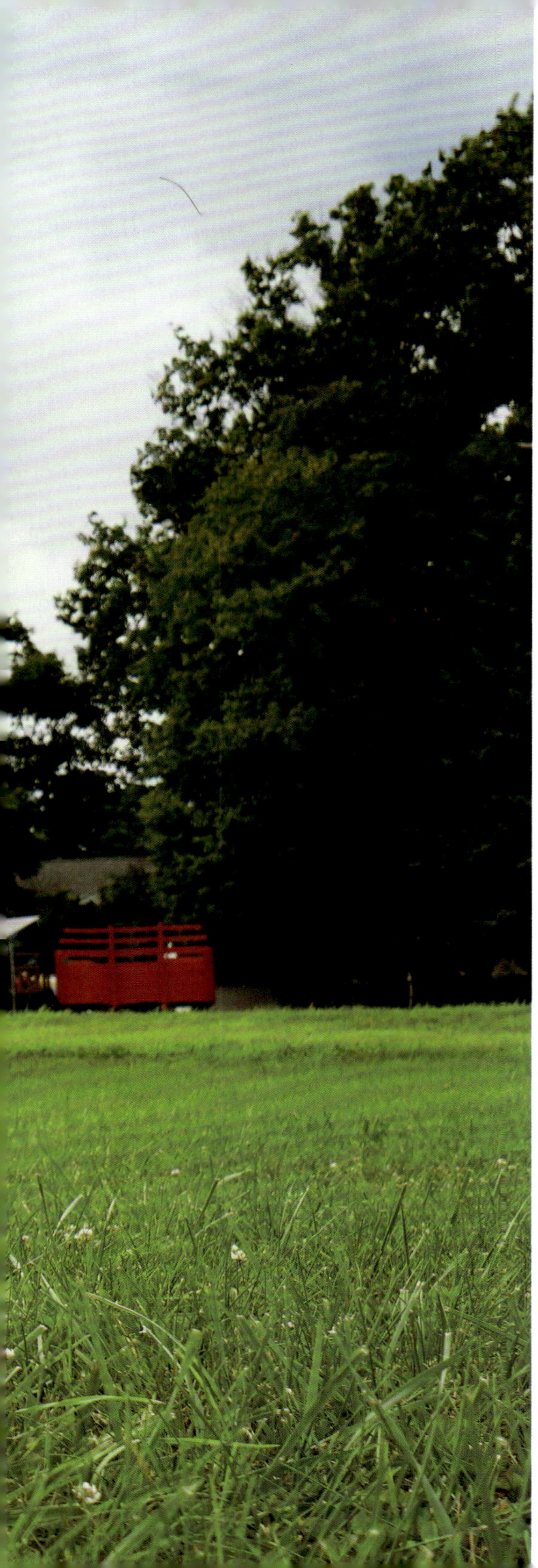

You can't help but think, "What if I did something differently? What if I changed my diet? What if I didn't eat that when I was pregnant?" But it wouldn't have mattered, because that had no bearing on any of it. It's just a lot of coping, like maybe I could change things, and just realizing that I can't change it, there's nothing I can do, so let's just do what we can.
– Jennifer, Addie's mother

Addie

Doctors predict that Addie, 4, who was diagnosed with a Related Intellectual Disability syndrome, will not exceed an IQ of 70. The genetic mutation, CTNNB1, prevents her body from making the protein necessary for neurological development. Addie was the 21st recorded case of this diagnosis. Addie is mostly nonverbal, not able to walk on her own, and is extremely farsighted. She has a feeding tube to help with her low weight and a communication device to help her express her needs. Addie loves to climb and bounce and is a huge fan of Mickey Mouse. Addie also loves to sing.

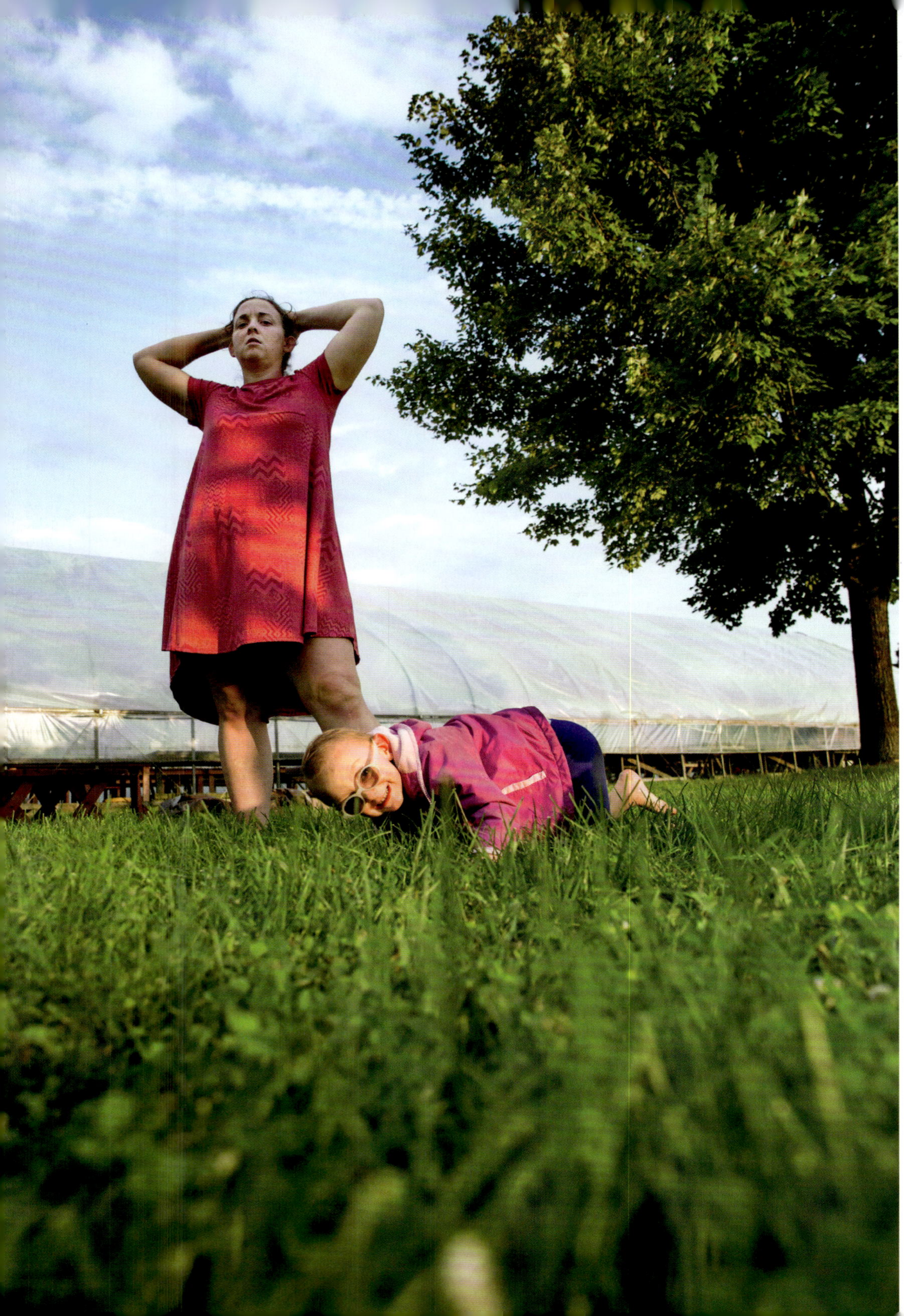

We had a lot of friends that had kids right at the same time, so we have a friend whose daughter is two days younger, we have someone a month older, two months younger. And now to see them all together and she's so far behind them. And so it's really, really hard when she is with the kids her own age because they still think she is a baby.
– Jennifer, Addie's mother

I think that's important to realize. We put so many labels, and you say, Okay, well this is where she should be. Just because these kids in the study didn't do it, doesn't mean she's not able to do it. It doesn't mean she can't. – Jennifer, Addie's mother

People say, "You know you've got to take care of yourself, too," and I think that's what falls by the wayside. You're so focused on making sure everything is okay here, that you forget. If she's going to be dependent on us for the rest of our lives, we've got to make sure that we're there for her. – Jennifer, Addie's mother

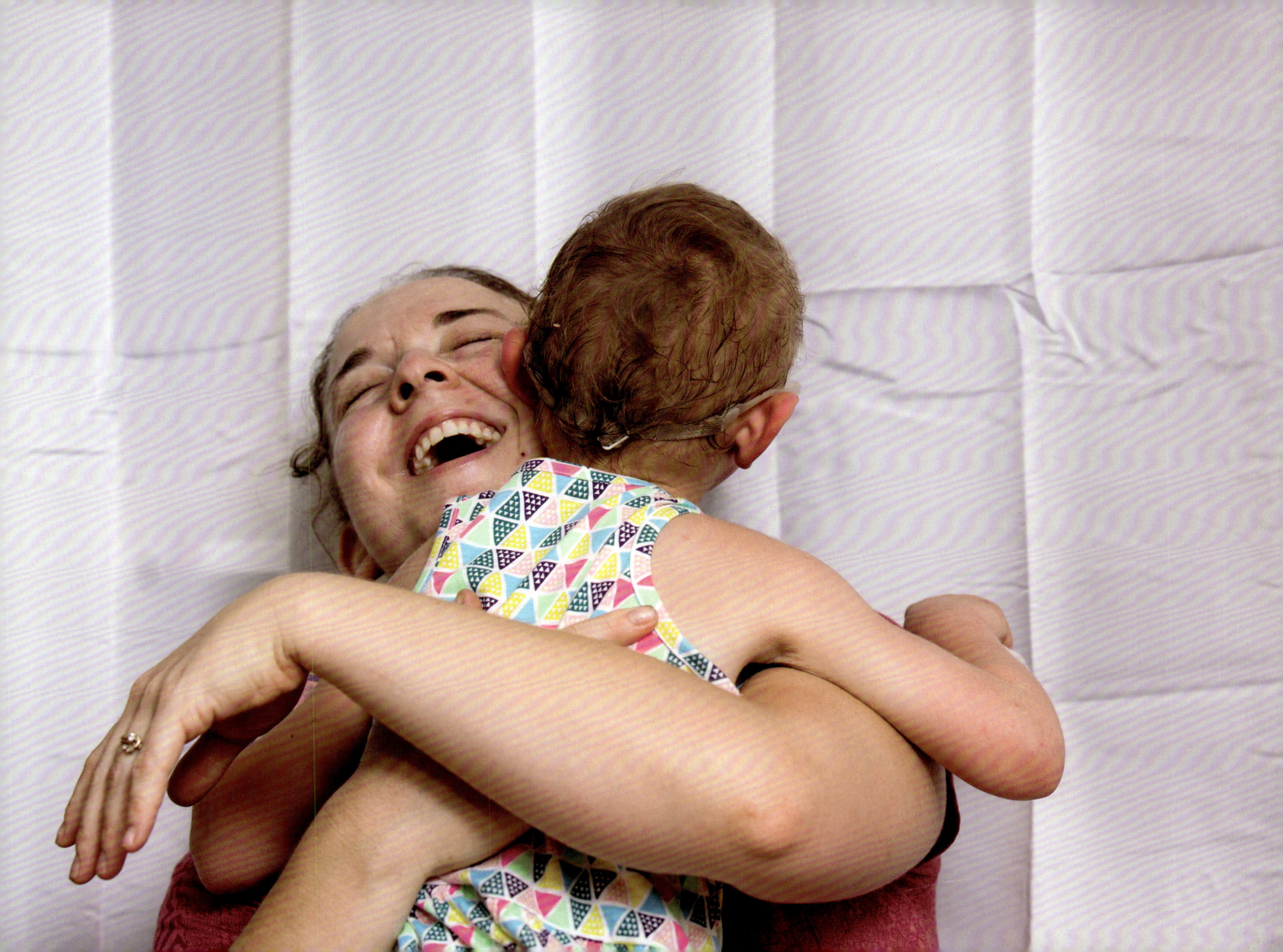

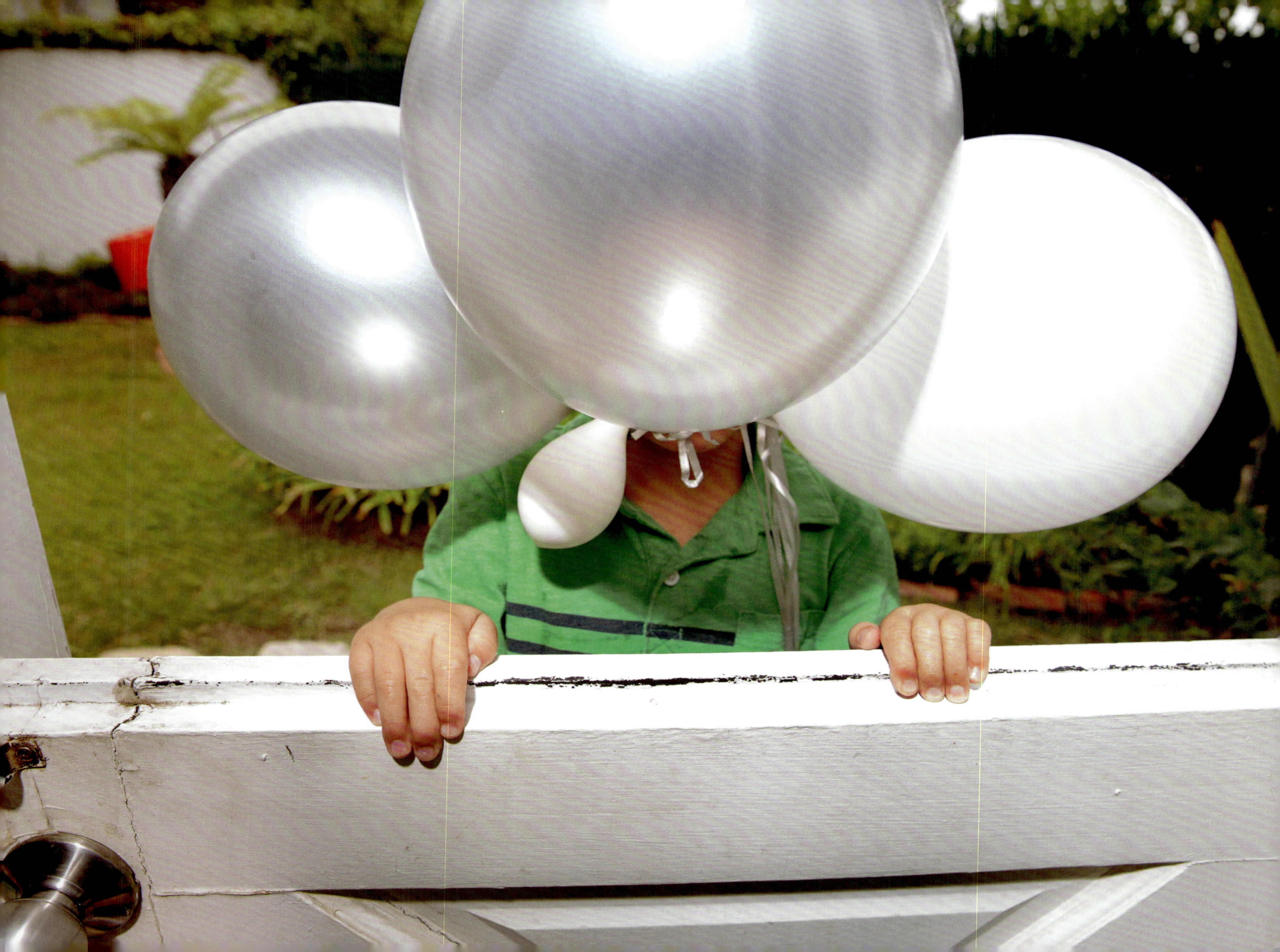

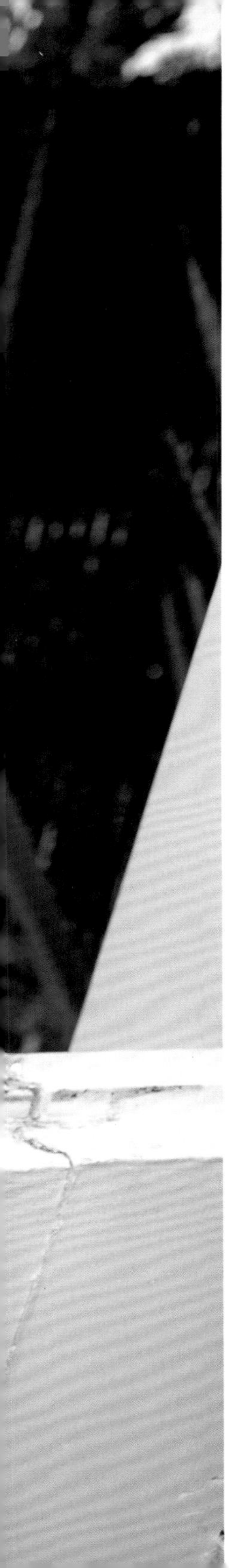

I always said when Ethan was diagnosed that we're not going to ever make a ceiling for him. He's going to get as far as he can, and our determination is just to make him the best Ethan he can be.
– Steph, Ethan's mom

Ethan

Ethan has two paternal 15th chromosomes, a rare form of a genetic disorder known as Angelman syndrome. Ethan does not sleep very much, has seizures, and can get frustrated when trying to communicate. His hands sometimes flap and he occasionally makes unexplained noises. Regardless of these symptoms, children with Angelman are known to have a generally happy demeanor. Ethan is no exception; he is constantly laughing, hugging, and smiling. Ethan loves water and playing with his brothers and on his iPad.

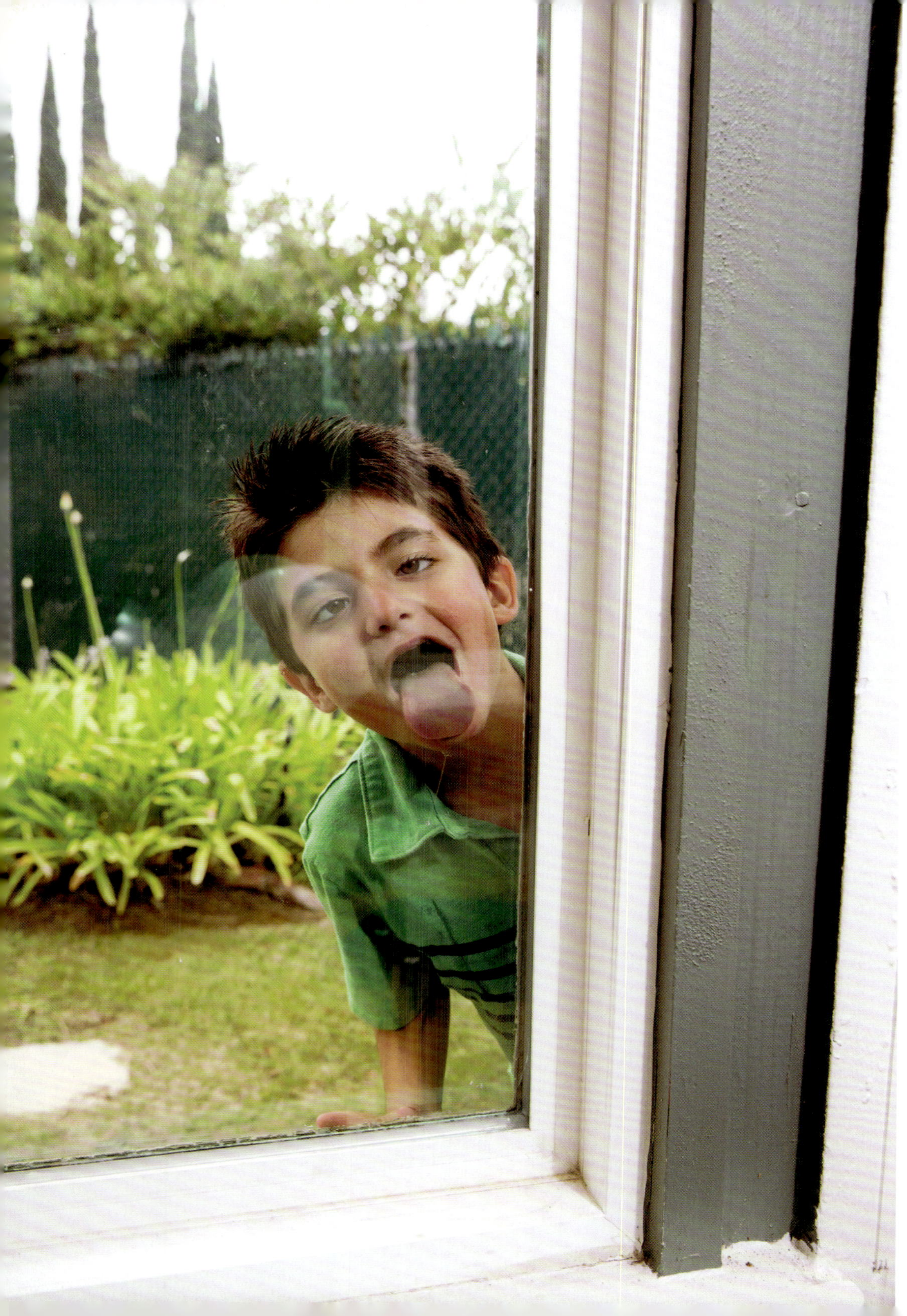

I've stopped caring what other people think around me because there's a lot of judgment from parents, especially ones that don't know. It doesn't look so good when you're dragging your kid out of a restaurant. It's not like he has a sign on that says, "I'm special needs and feel bad for my mom," or, "Don't judge her."
– Steph, Ethan's mom

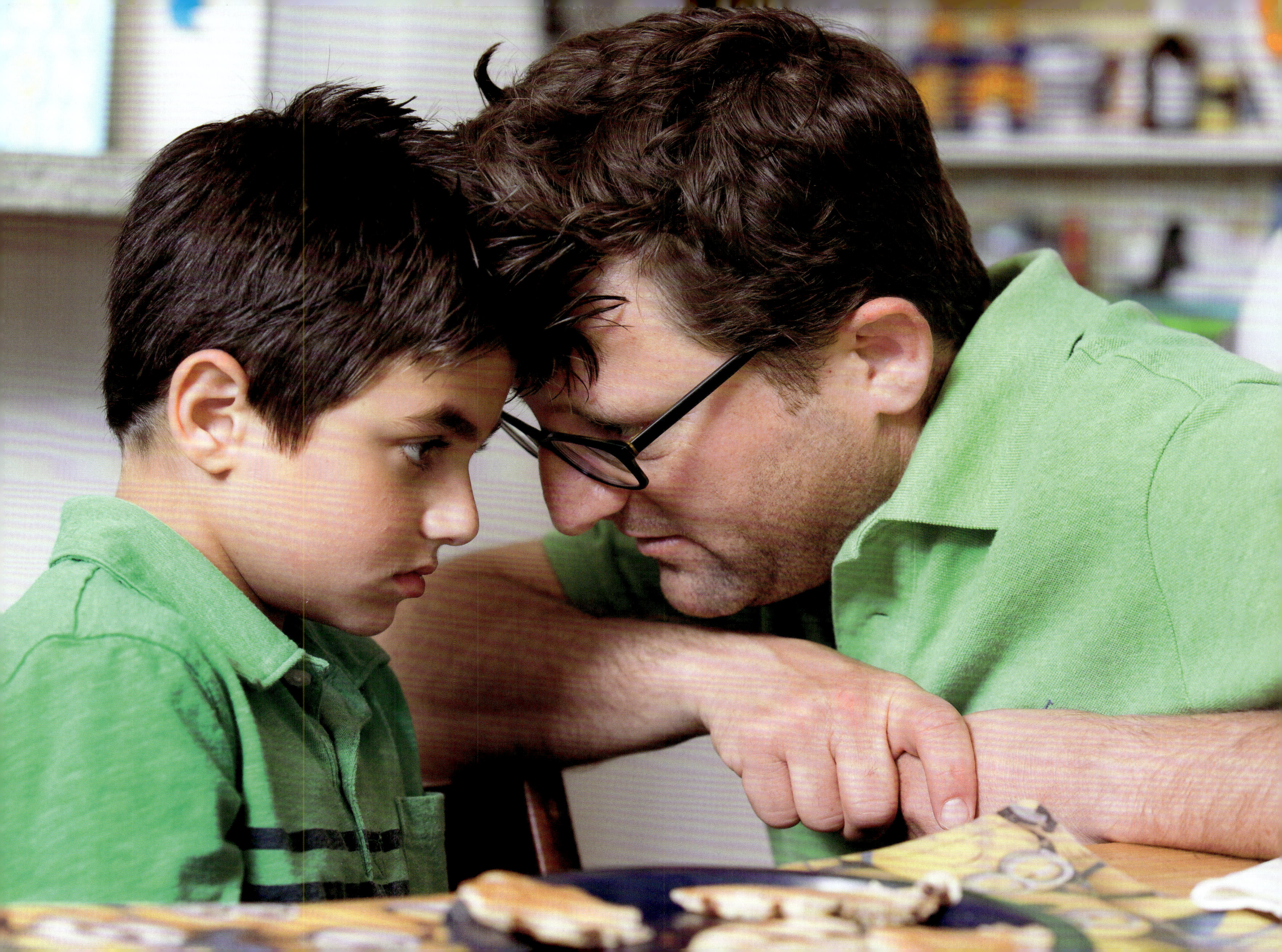

I think that watching him have seizures was probably one of the most painful experiences as a parent, because you're helpless. You just have to ride it out, and there's absolutely nothing you can do.
– Steph, Ethan's mother

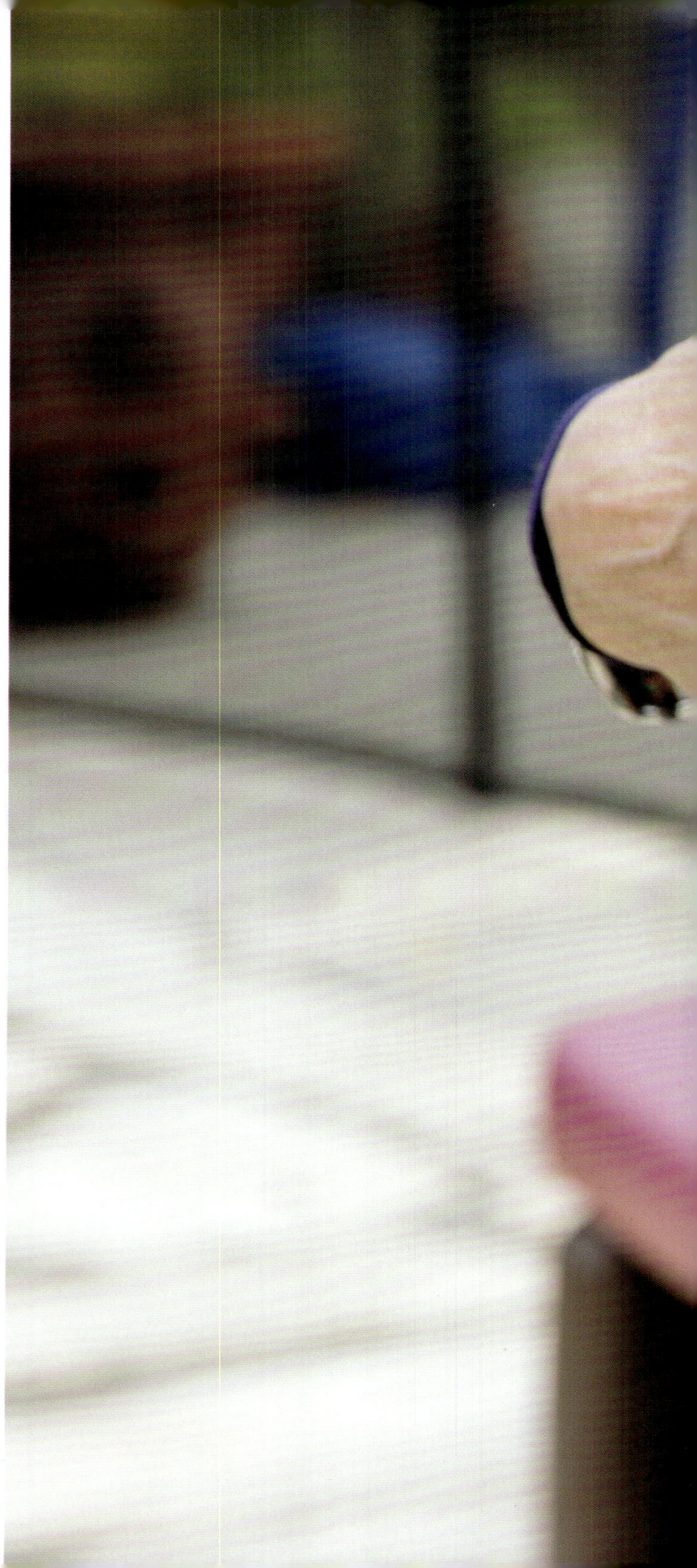

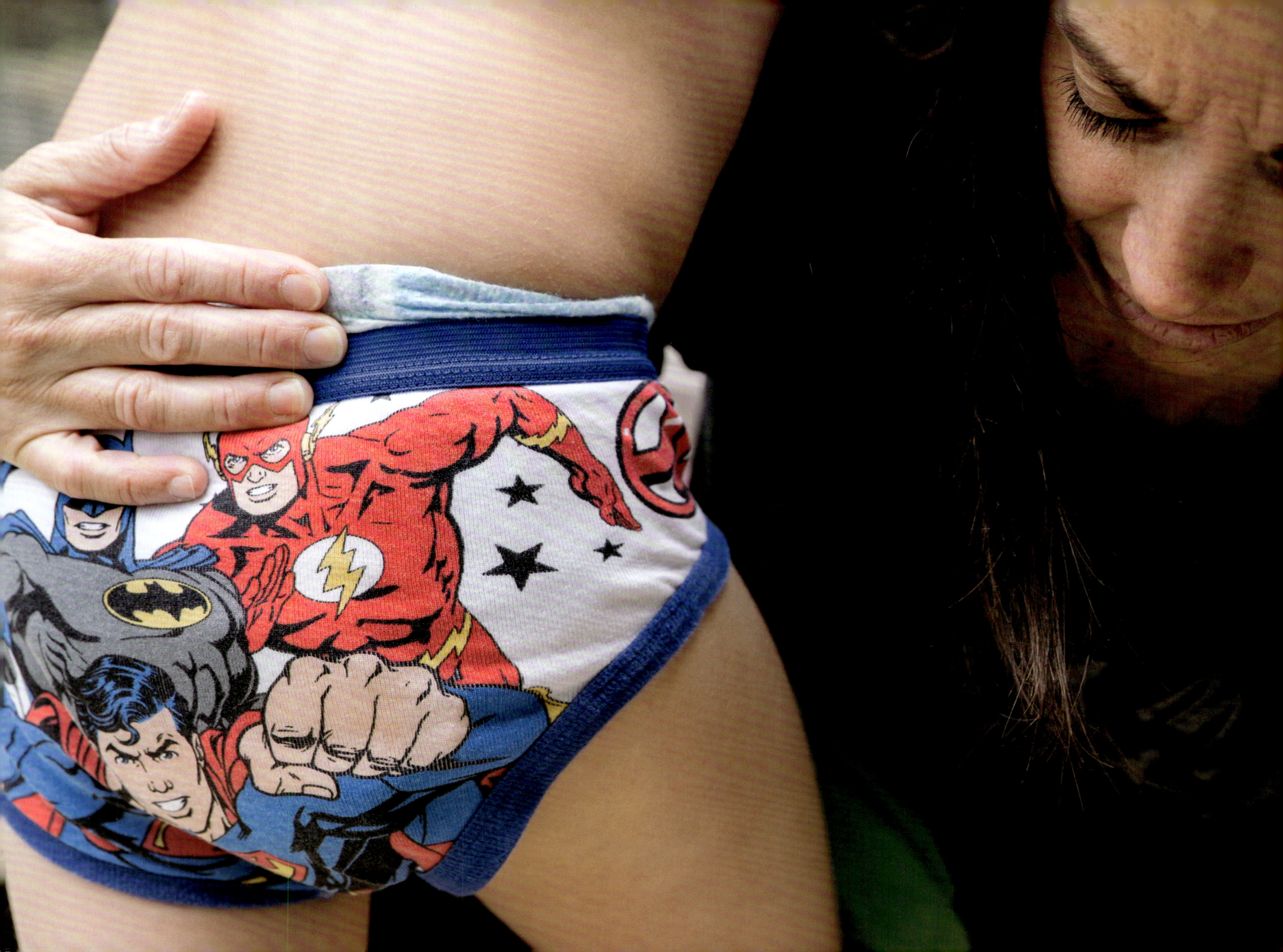

I've learned a lot about not judging people without knowing them. I've had to be more patient which is a good quality to have. It's hard when he gets aggressive and stuck or breaks my stuff. He gives the best hugs and has the cutest smile. – Zach, Ethan's brother

Having a brother like Ethan is like sort of a rose. Some days are like petals, beautiful and nice, and other days are thorny and hard to handle. In the end, you love the whole rose and all it's parts. – Josh, Ethan's brother

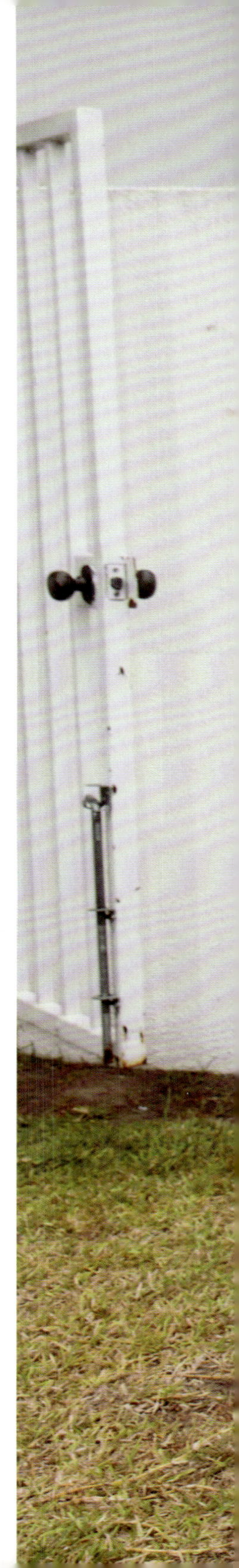

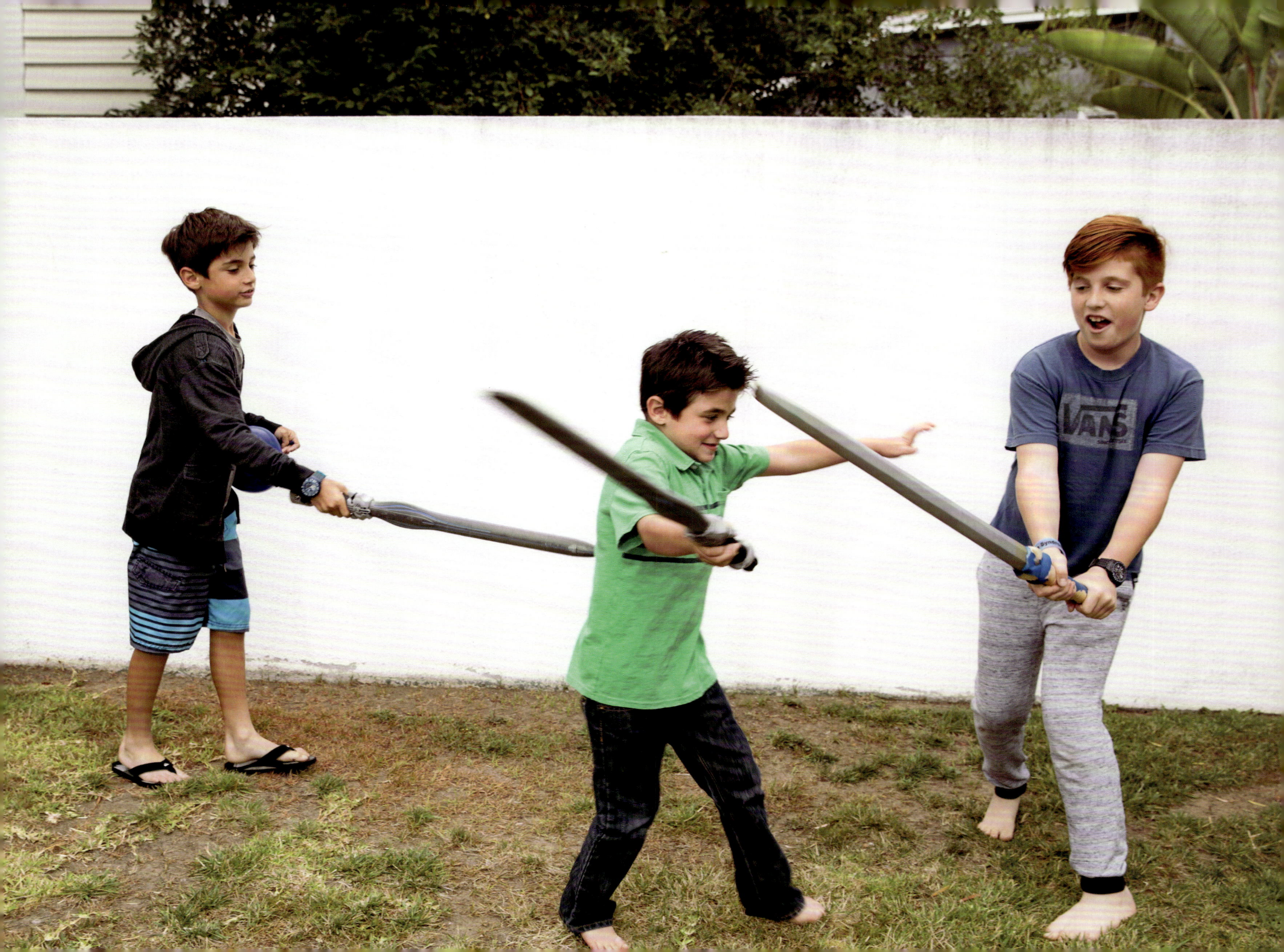
VANS

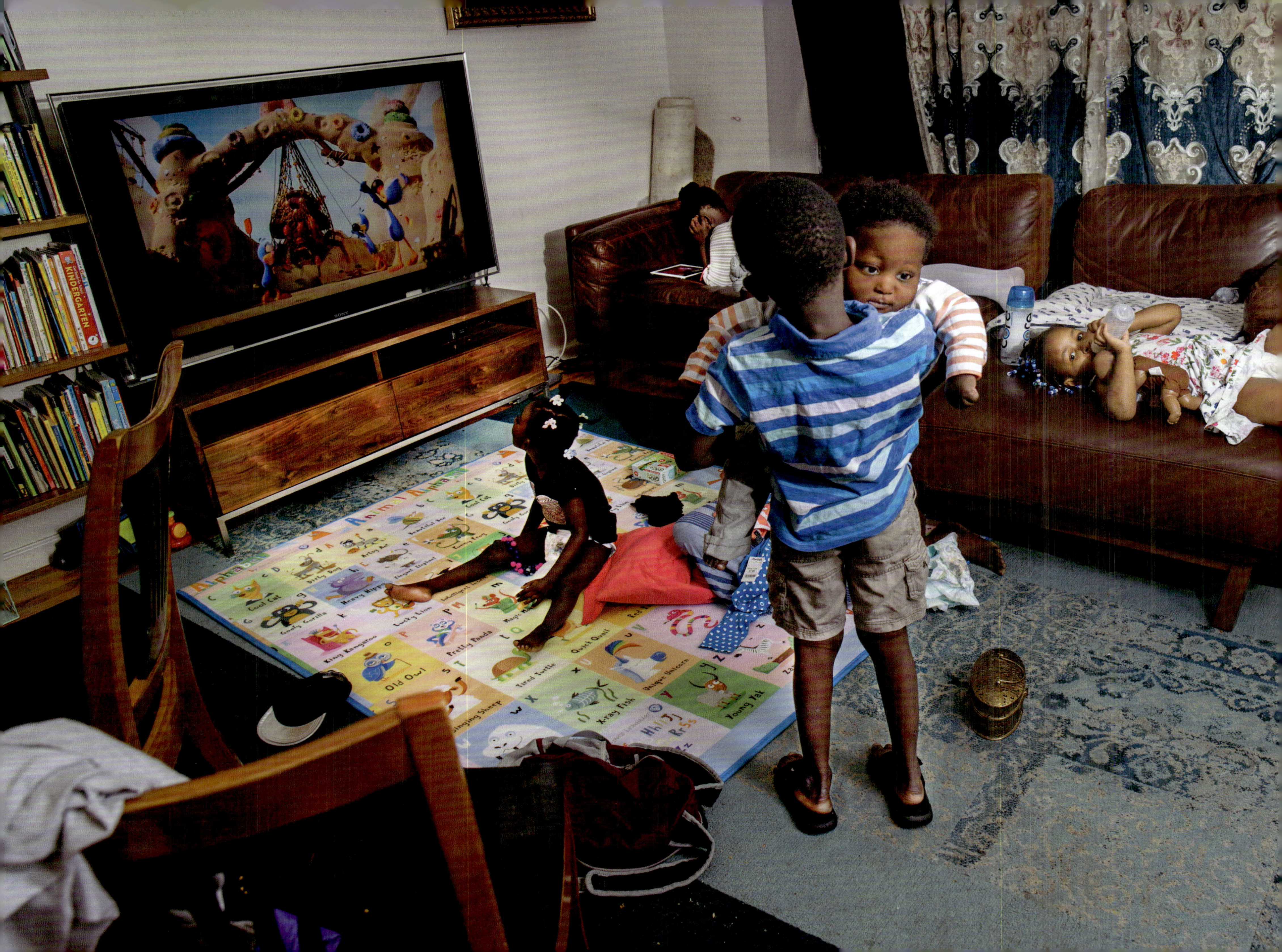
KINDERGARTEN
Cool Cat
Goofy Gorilla
Heavy Hippo
King Kangaroo
Old Owl
Pretty Panda
Quick Quail
Tired Turtle
Unique Unicorn
X-ray Fish
Young Yak
Singing Sheep

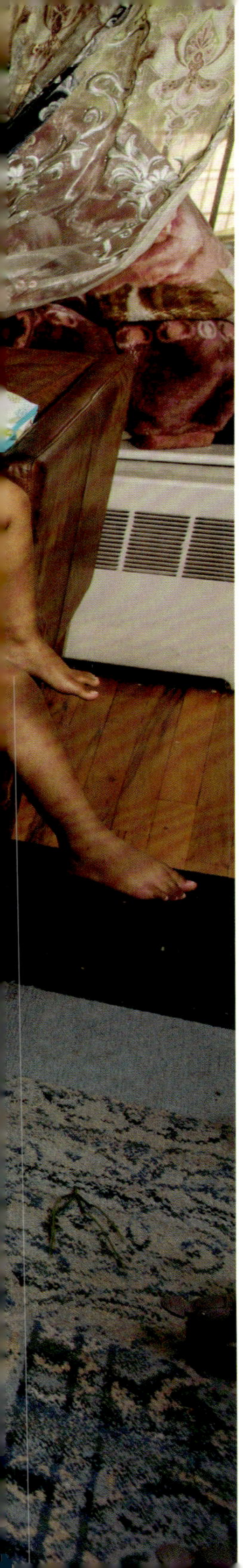

Shortly after Mohammed was born, I got Miriam's diagnosis—NGLY1. As I was about to hang up the phone the doctor told me that my newborn son Mohammed has it too.
– Ami, Miriam and Mohammed's mother

KIDS WITH RARE CONDITIONS OFTEN REQUIRE THE ASSISTANCE OF YOUNG SIBLINGS. ALEJANDRE, AGE 5, HOLDS HIS BABY BROTHER.

Miriam & Mohammed

Miriam and Mohammed are the first black children diagnosed with NGLY1, and Mohammed is the youngest ever. There are 30 known cases in the world. Symptoms include developmental delays, liver dysfunction, smaller head, diminished reflexes, seizures, and lack of tears—among others. The diagnoses for both of Amientabah's children came in the same phone call, just days after Mohammed's birth.

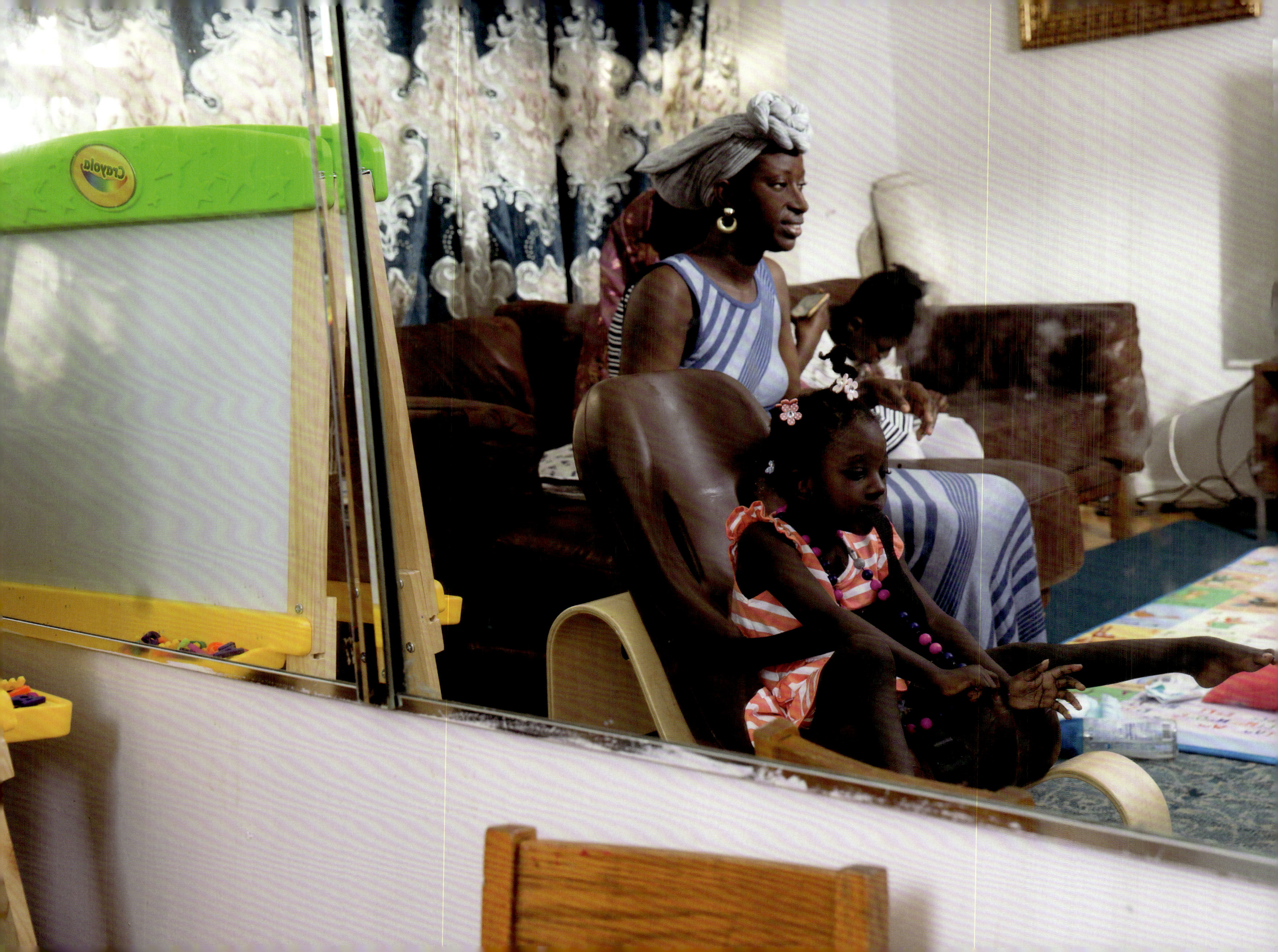

People kept telling me, some kids are slower than the other kids. It will come. But I knew something was wrong with my child, and I sat down on the Internet late in the night doing research. What are you going to do if you have a child who's slow and who is weak? – *Ami, Miriam and Mohammed's mother*

I went to a geneticist, Joya, because I wanted to know what my child had because I felt the guilt. They said if I wanted to do a test, I have to pay $12,000. I didn't have money. So I had a goal to save money by the time she turned three. I had saved $8,000 when Joya called and said: "My mentor at New York-Presbyterian said he is willing to do volunteer work and test Miriam." That's one of the happiest moments—I cried, because knowing what your child has, is just a relief of burden. I mean, if you know, you can help. – Ami, Miriam and Mohammed's mother

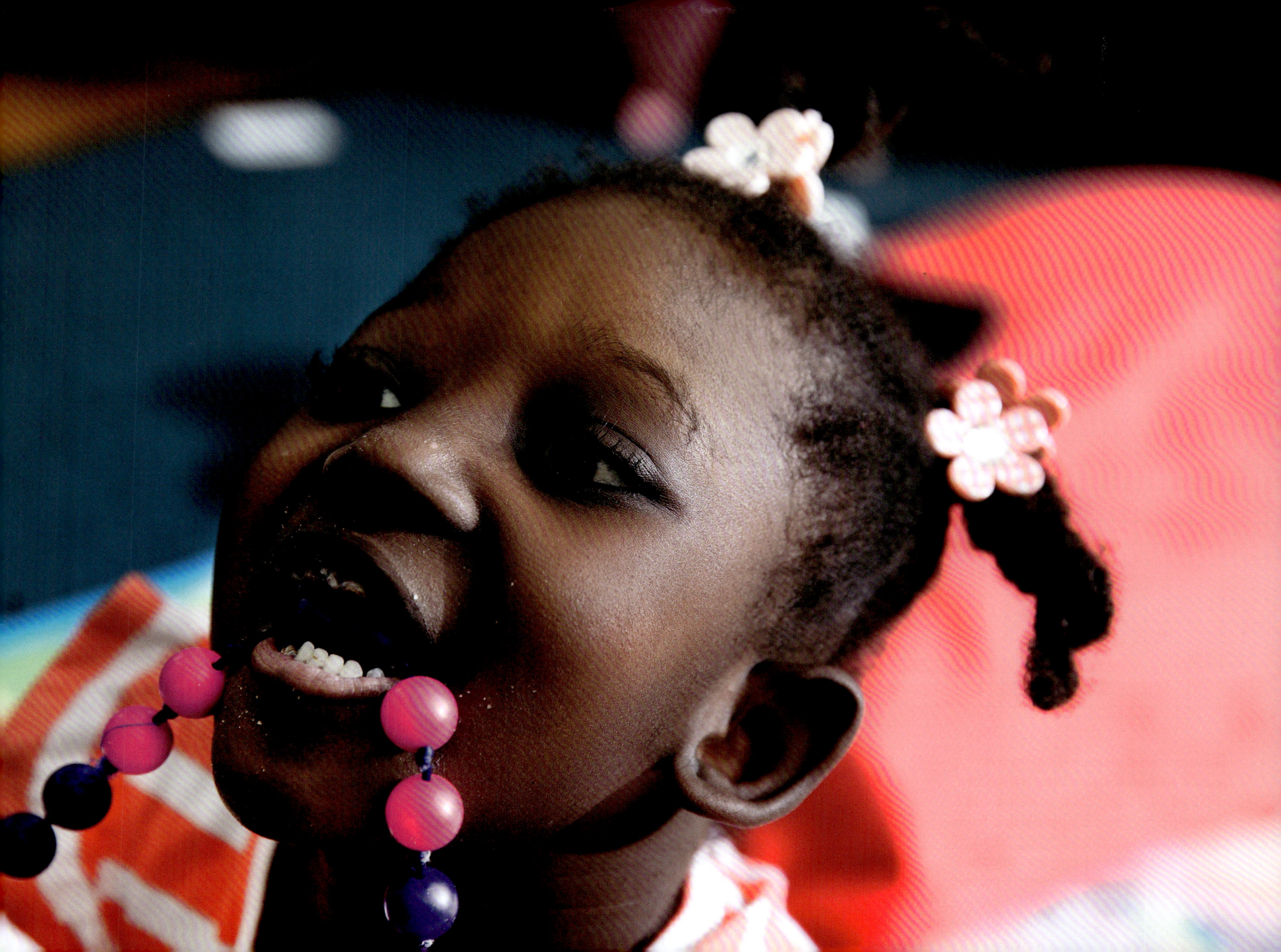

MIRIAM AND MOHAMMED'S EYES DON'T PRODUCE TEARS AND THEY MUST USE DROPS TO AVOID PAIN, ULCERS AND SCARS ON THE CORNEA, WHICH CAN CAUSE BLINDNESS.

Miriam and Mohammed's mom was pained that she couldn't breastfeed her children. She says, "I was grieving and I was criticized from my people and from their dad saying that I'm being a horrible mother not breastfeeding my children."
– Ami, Miriam and Mohammed's mother

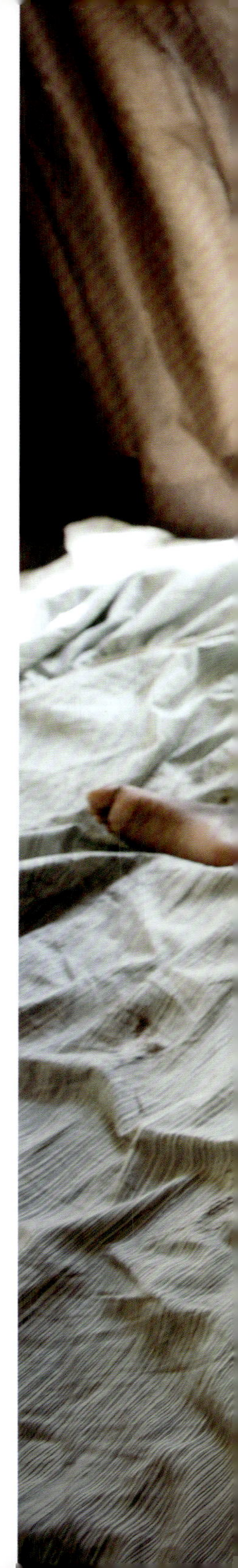

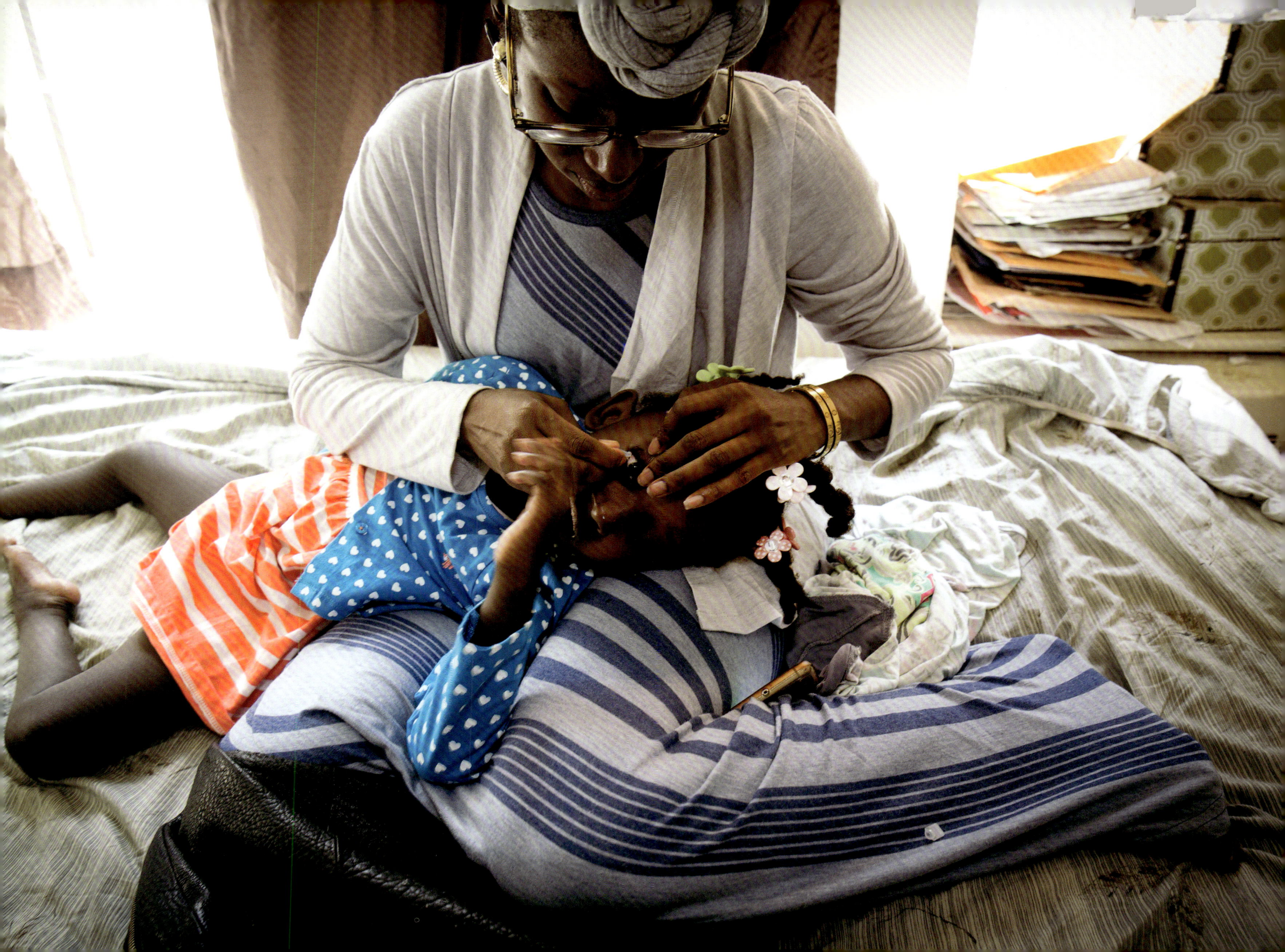

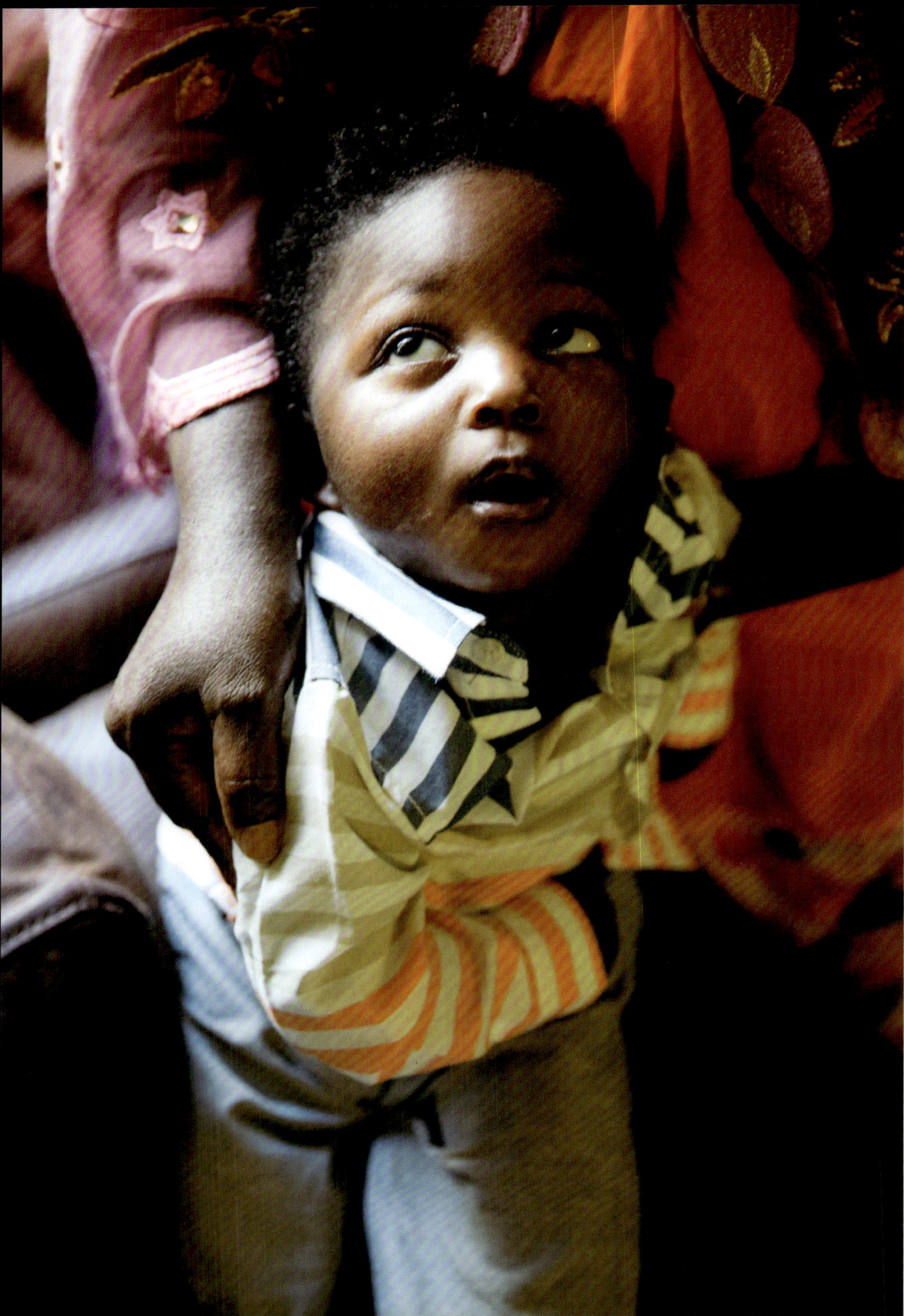

I worry about them. What about society? How will they join them? What about if I'm not here? We live in a world where people are more likely to judge you than opening their heart. And I'm worried about how people are going to treat them because they're vulnerable.
– Ami, Miriam and Mohammed's mother

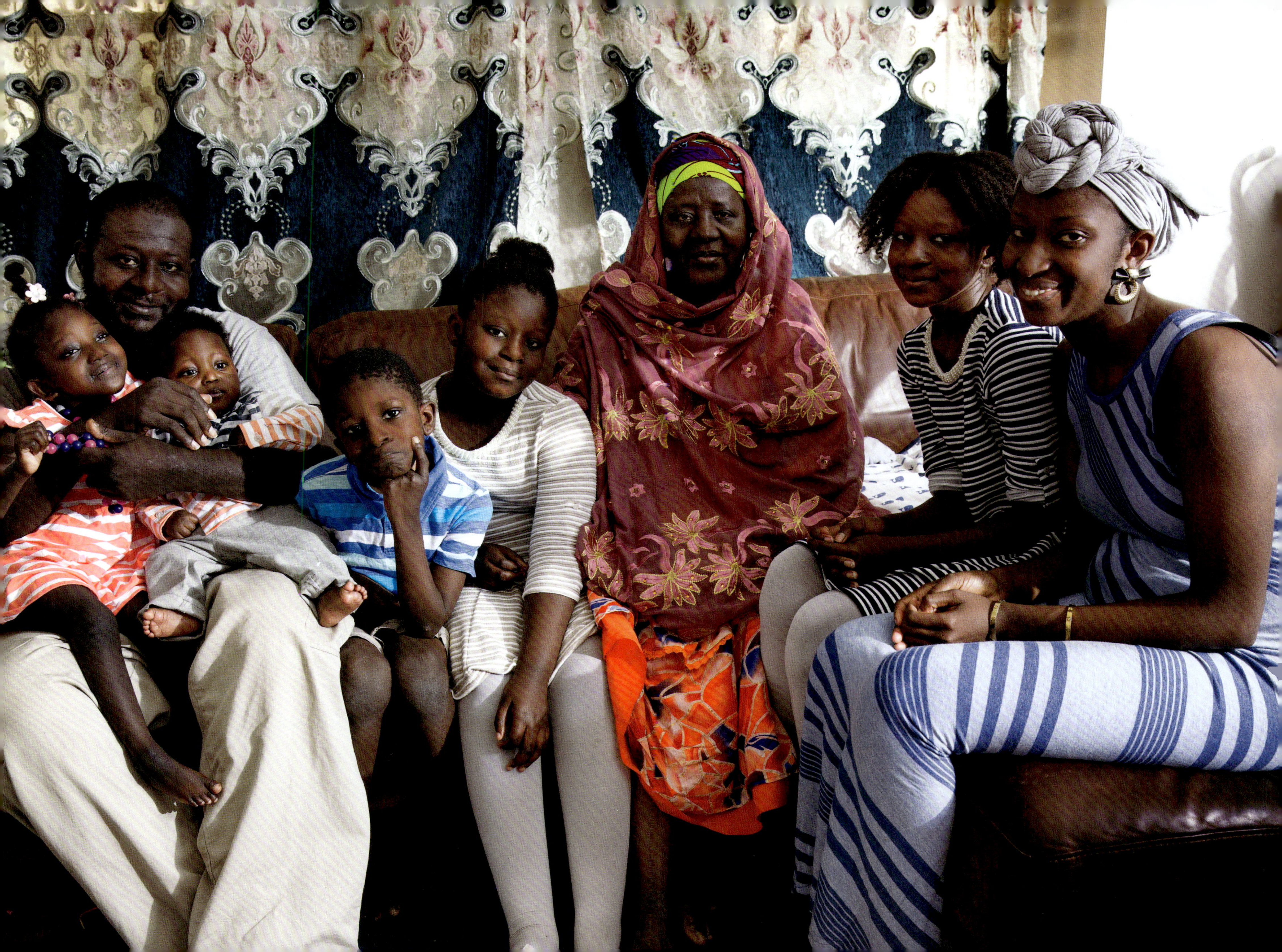

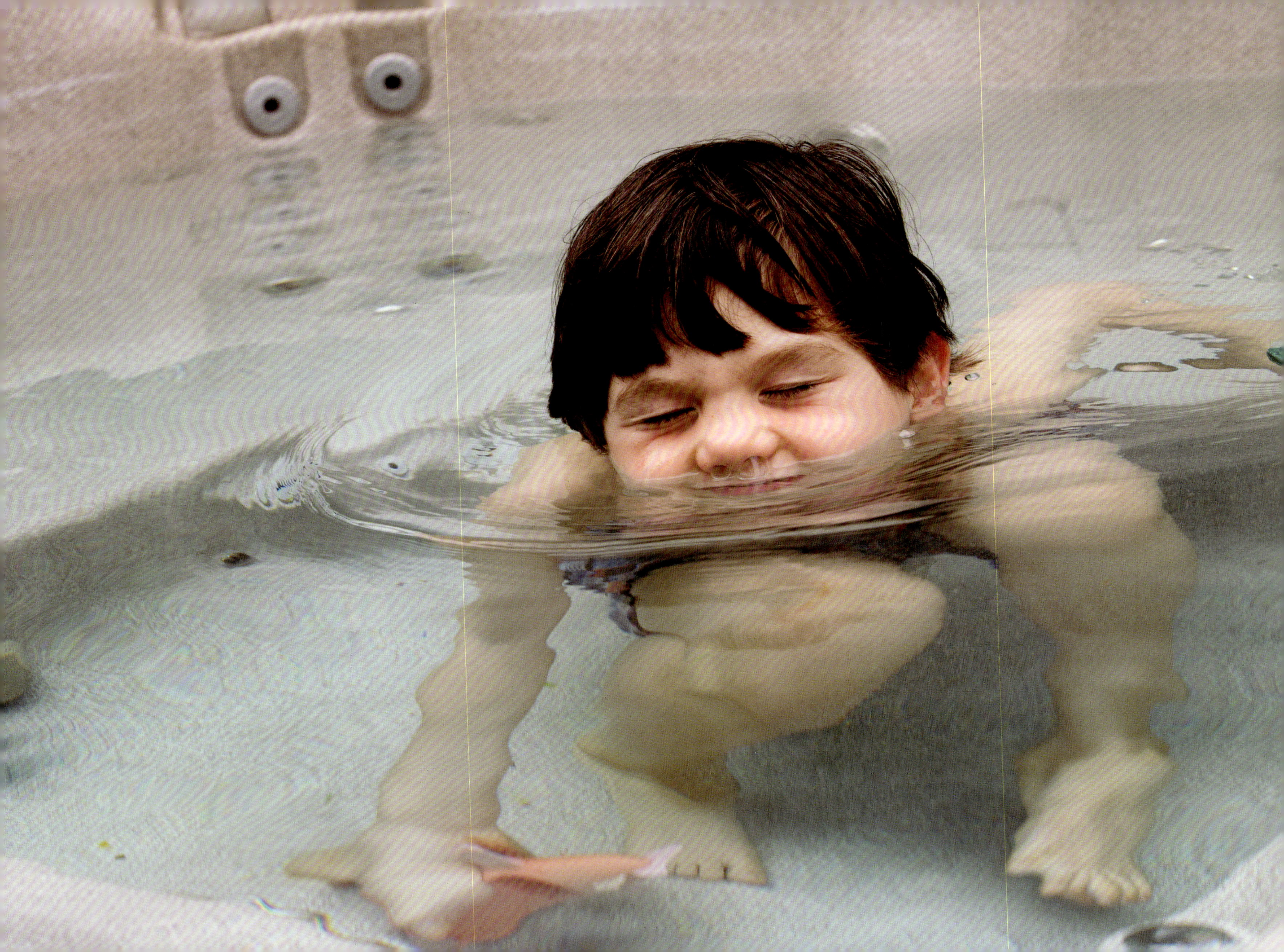

It's one thing to say, "Hey we support you," but I don't think anyone truly appreciates what we go through on a daily basis. – Jonas, Darus's father

Darus

Darus's parents first grew concerned when their son reached the age of two. Insurance denied the request for an exome sequencing test three times. Eventually, the state covered the costs, and the test discovered a genetic mutation known as Phelan-McDermid syndrome. Darus is not able to feed himself, dress himself, use the bathroom himself, or verbally express the way he feels. He is in near-constant motion and has little to no sense of fear or danger. Darus loves playing at the beach and watching garbage trucks.

You think you could bring a 5-year-old to a movie, but that's not even a possibility in our world. I guess it's multiple frustrations that we feel—little pieces at a time. Whether it's going to a kid's birthday party or going to a family function, we can never really relax, there's always constant vigilance required in order to make sure he's not getting into something he shouldn't be into.
–Jonas, Darus's father

DARUS'S PARENTS HAVE A VISUAL WARNING FOR MOTORISTS SINCE HE OFTEN RUNS OUT OF THEIR SIGHT.

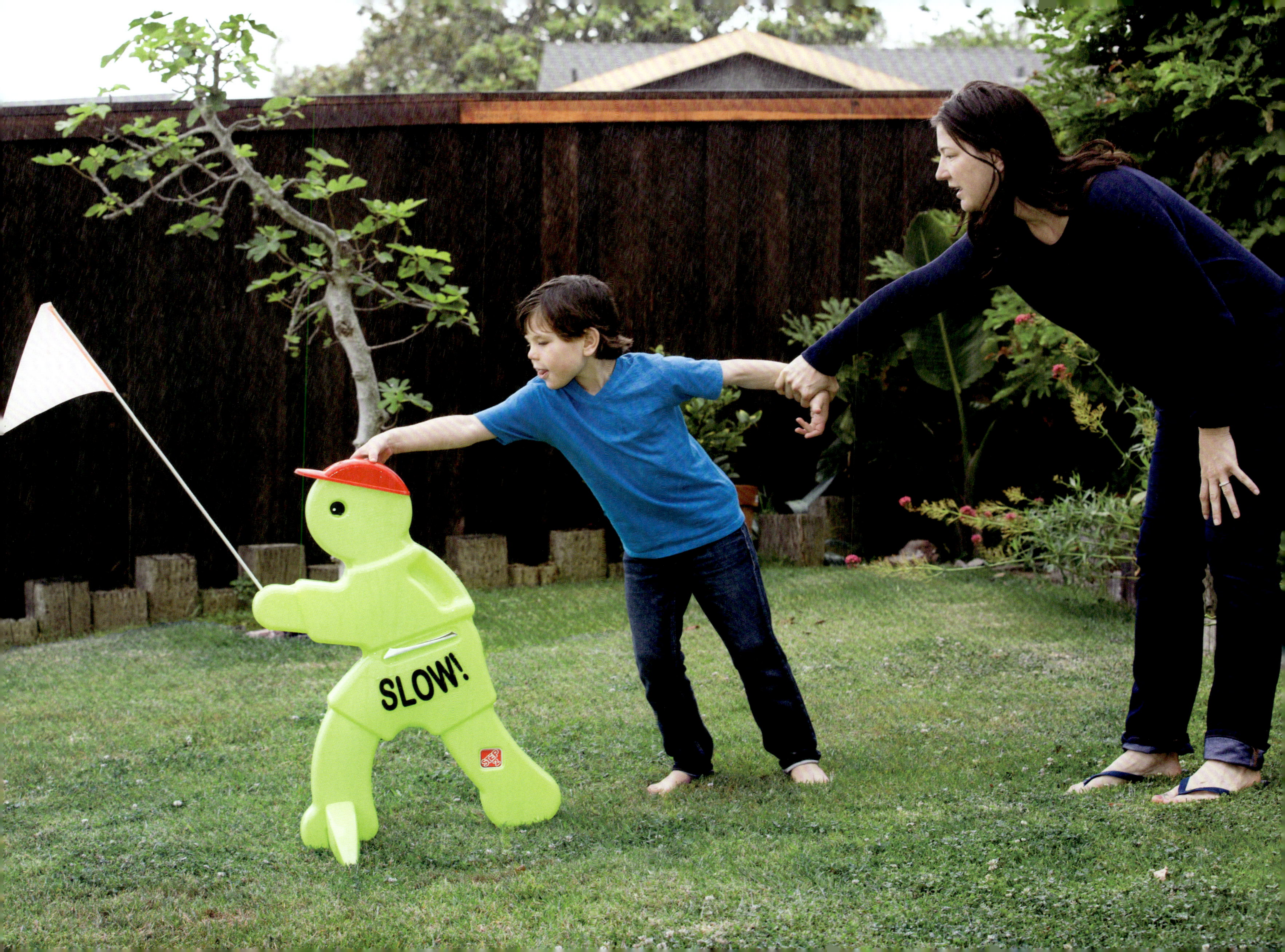
SLOW!

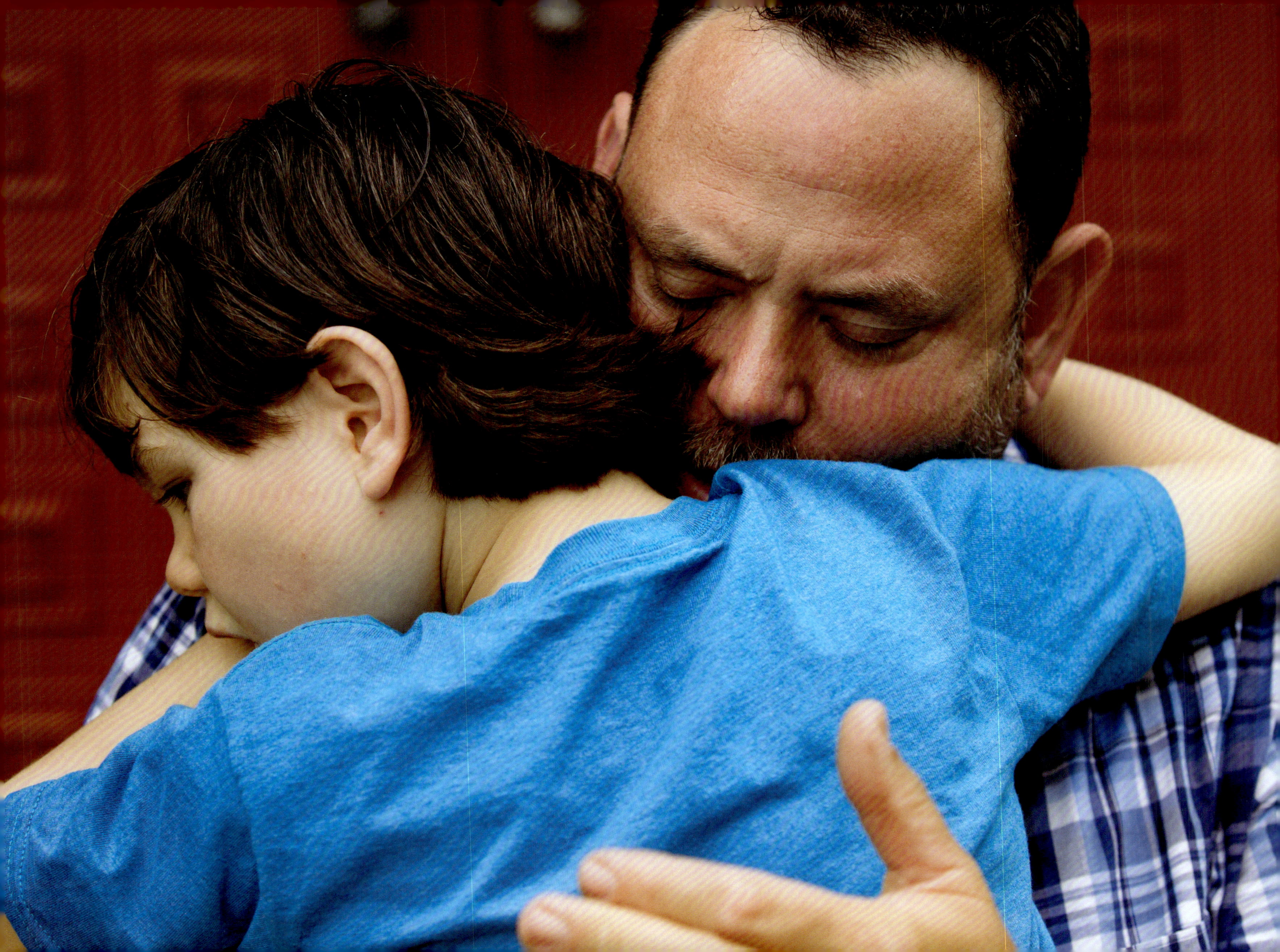

There have been some letdowns. I also think some people just don't know what to do, or how to help. Sometimes we just have to be direct and let them know. But Darus has given us a lot of gifts: compassion, empathy, and understanding, to name a few.
– Abby, Darus's mother

She brightens up the room with her big beautiful eyes and smile. We love to play with her and hear her infectious belly laugh. We just have to appreciate every moment because we don't know how long we have before she starts to lose the skills she has gained. It is extremely heartbreaking for our whole family to realize how devastating this disorder BPAN is and what will happen in the future. – Jennifer, Madison's mother

Madison

It took Madison's family two and a half years to get answers. Finally, whole exome sequencing revealed a rare degenerative progressive disorder known as beta-propeller protein-associated neurodegeneration (BPAN), a neurodegeneration with brain iron accumulation (NBIA) disorder. Madison, 3, cannot walk or speak, has intellectual disability, poor motor planning, sleep disorder, and suffers from seizures. This disorder is frequently associated with the eventual development of dystonia, dementia, Parkinson's, blindness, and premature loss of life. Madison loves music, turning pages in a book, and tapping blocks together. Her favorite activity is going on the swings.

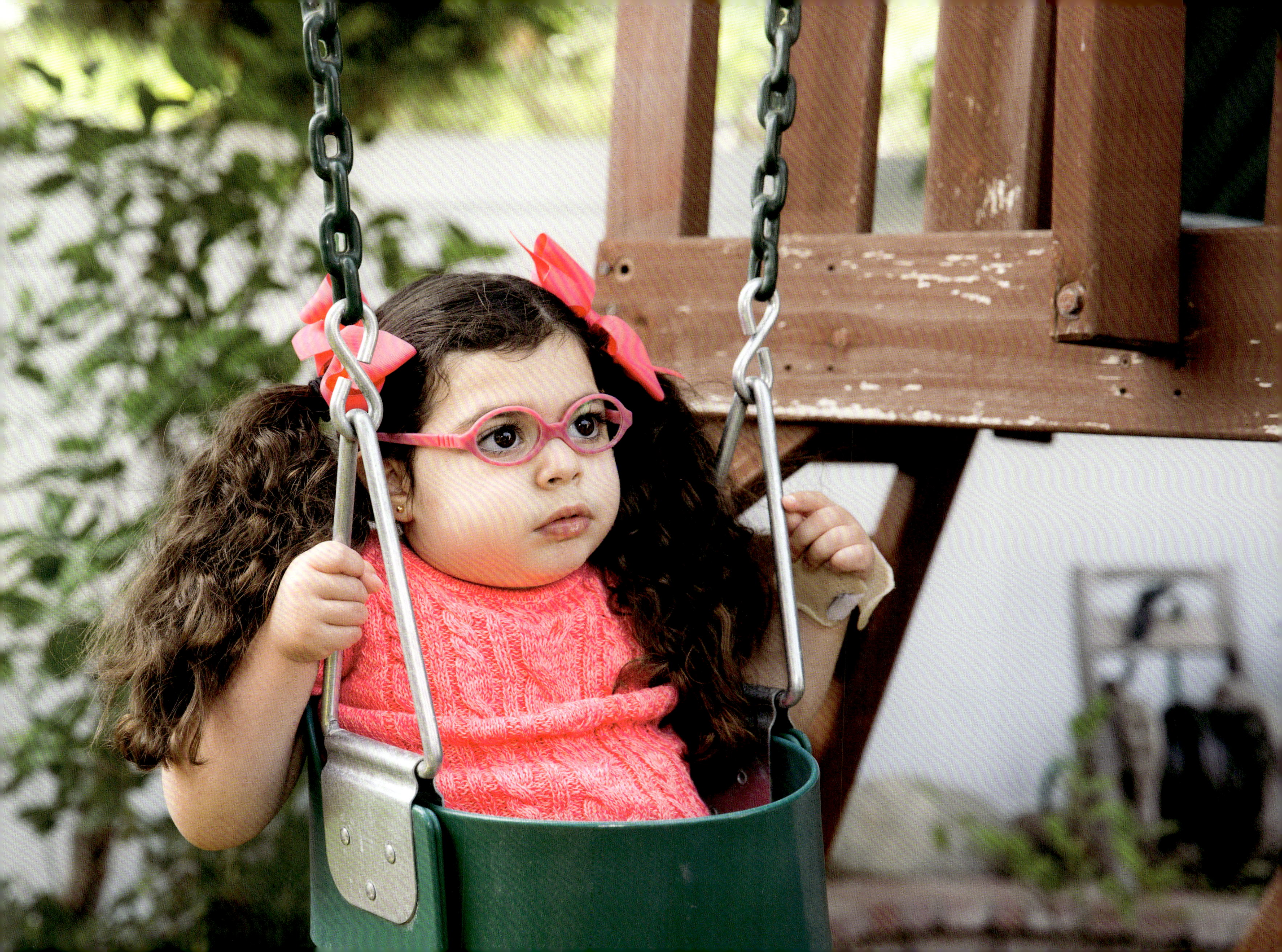

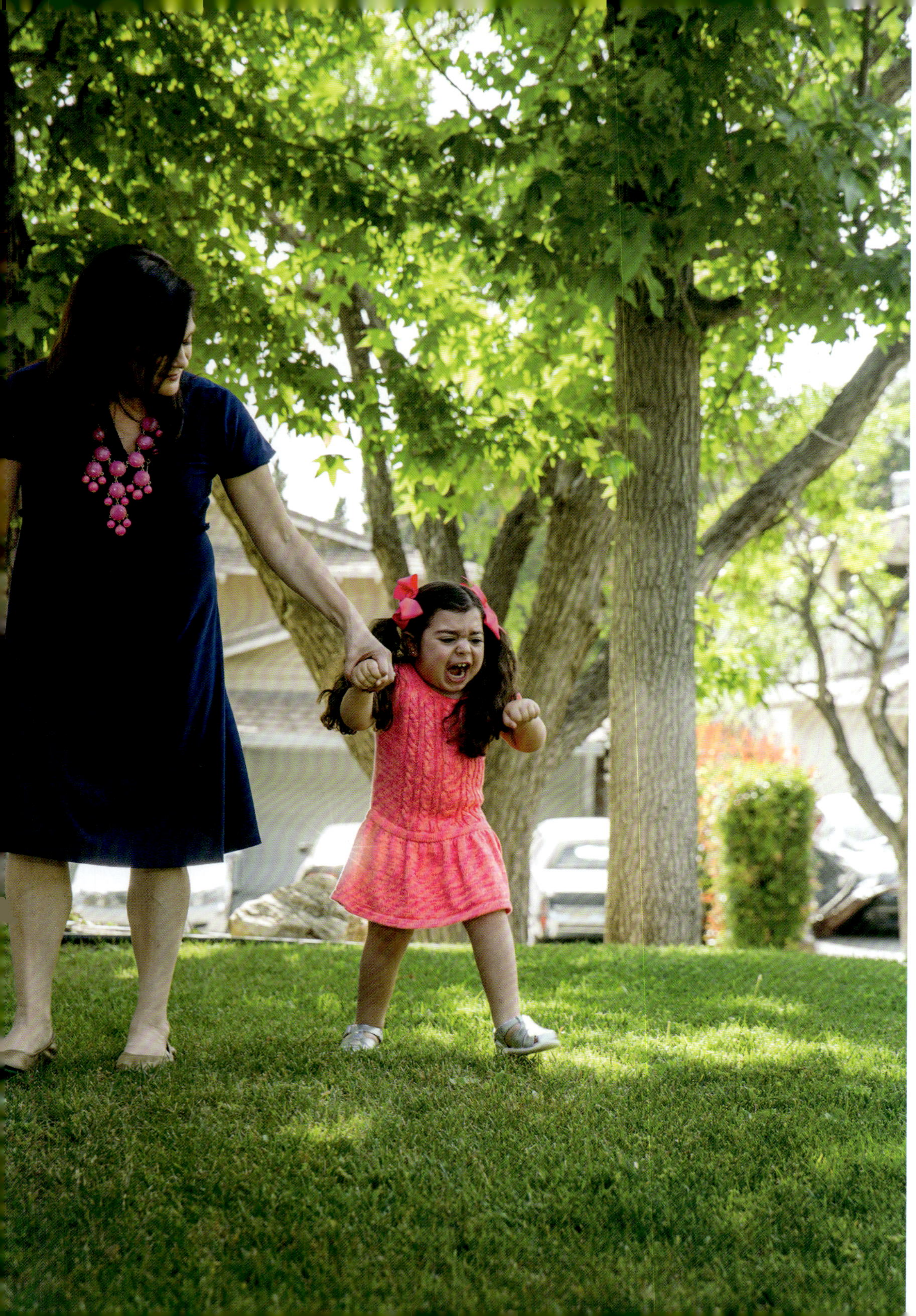

My goal is to bring awareness for this new disorder that is very rare around the world. It's so rare that there are approximately 100 people in the whole world who are registered to have this. There could be hundreds of more kids who have BPAN but they just haven't been diagnosed.
– Jennifer, Madison's mother

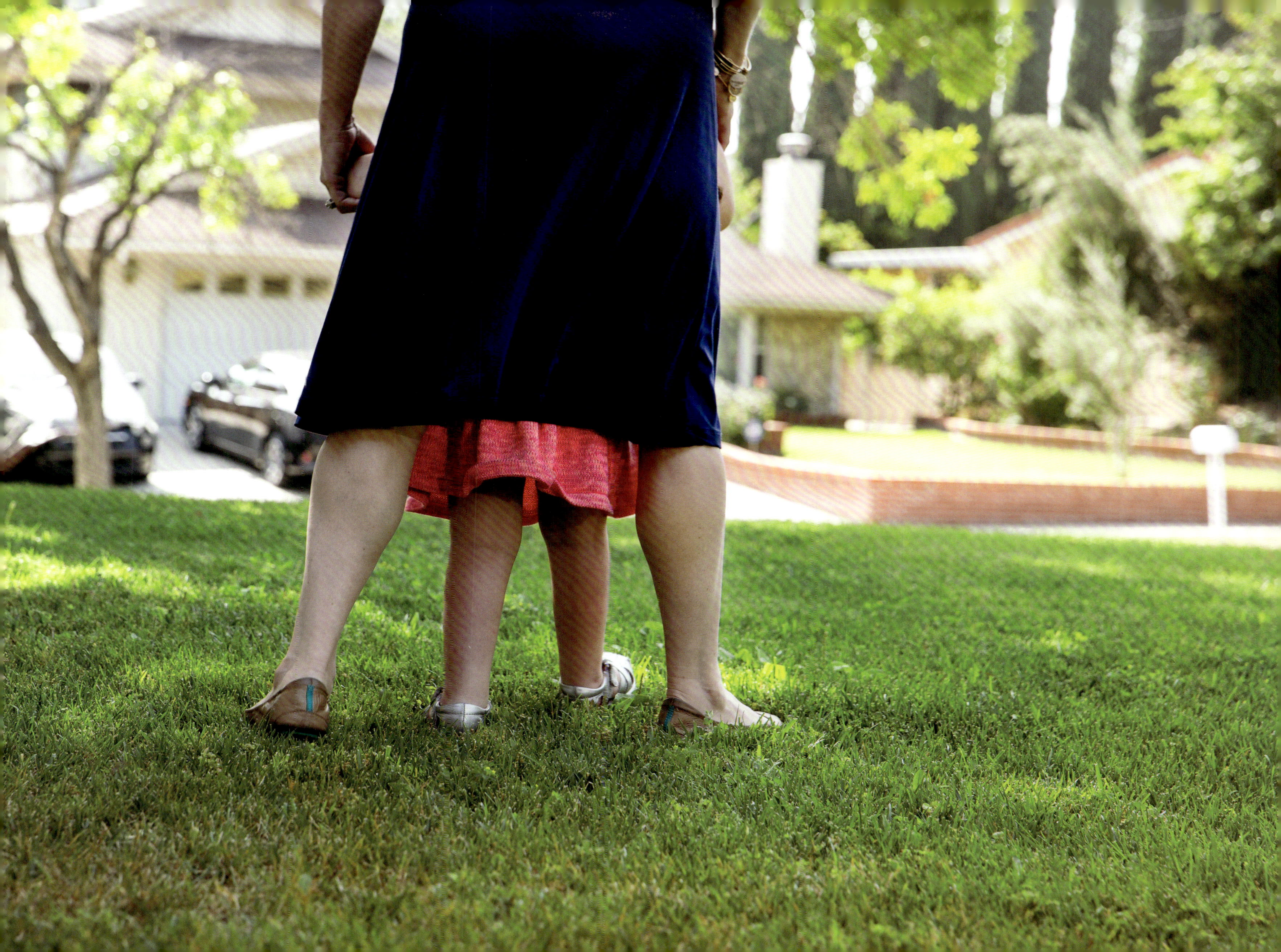

LOUIS'S SKIN STRETCHES AN ABNORMAL AMOUNT DUE TO HIS CONDITION.

Louis

It took three years and two geneticists for Louis to receive his diagnosis—Ehlers-Danlos syndrome, Postural Orthostatic Tachycardia Syndrome, and dysautonomia. He was not diagnosed until the age of 12. As a result of his conditions, Louis's heart rate falls dangerously low, causing what he describes as a "crash." Overcome by dizziness and lightheadedness, Louis has to immediately stop what he is doing. He has gastrointestinal problems and his joints sublux and dislocate randomly. Louis, 15, loves to joke around and hang out with his friends. He has been drumming since second grade but now struggles to focus when playing.

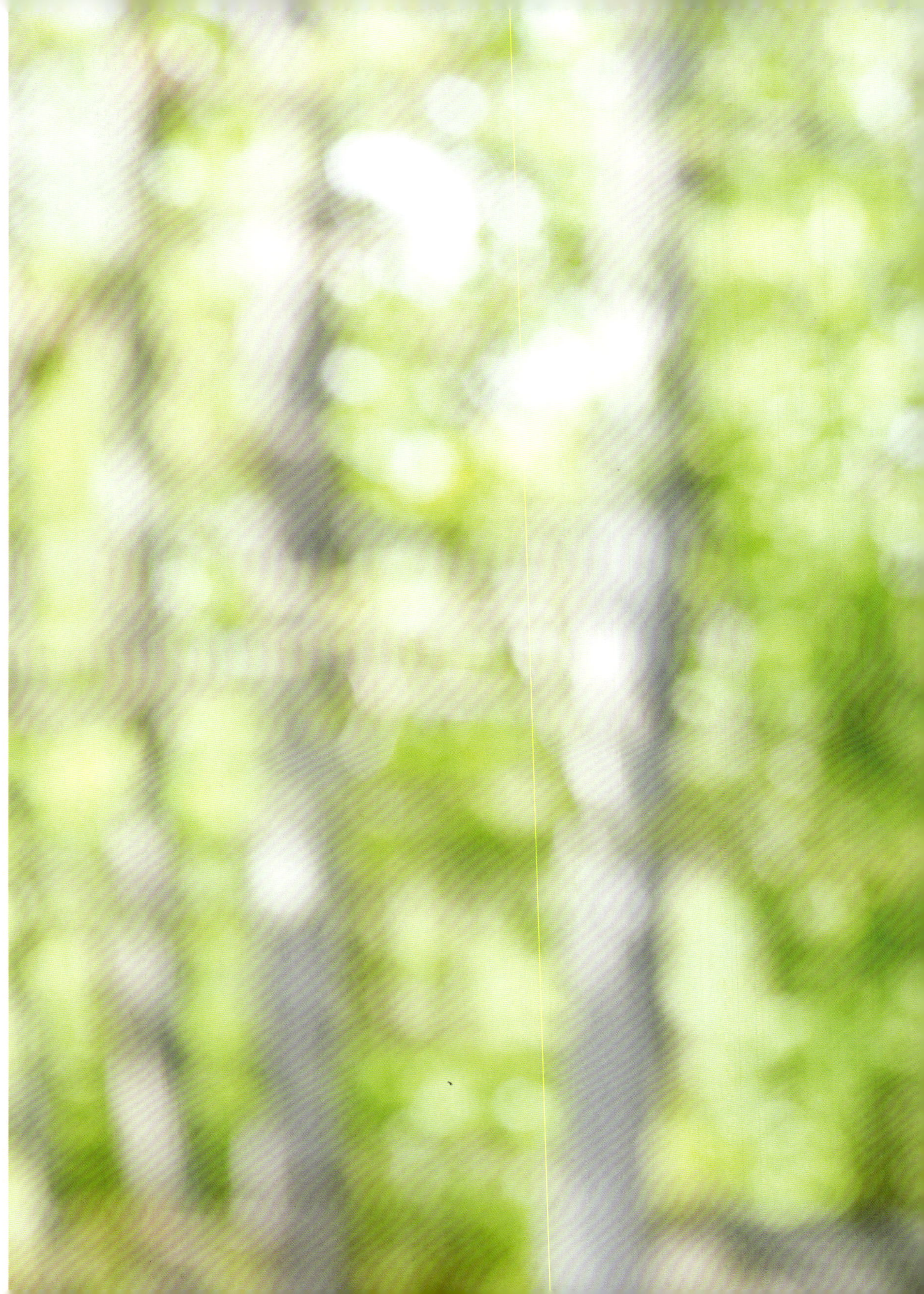

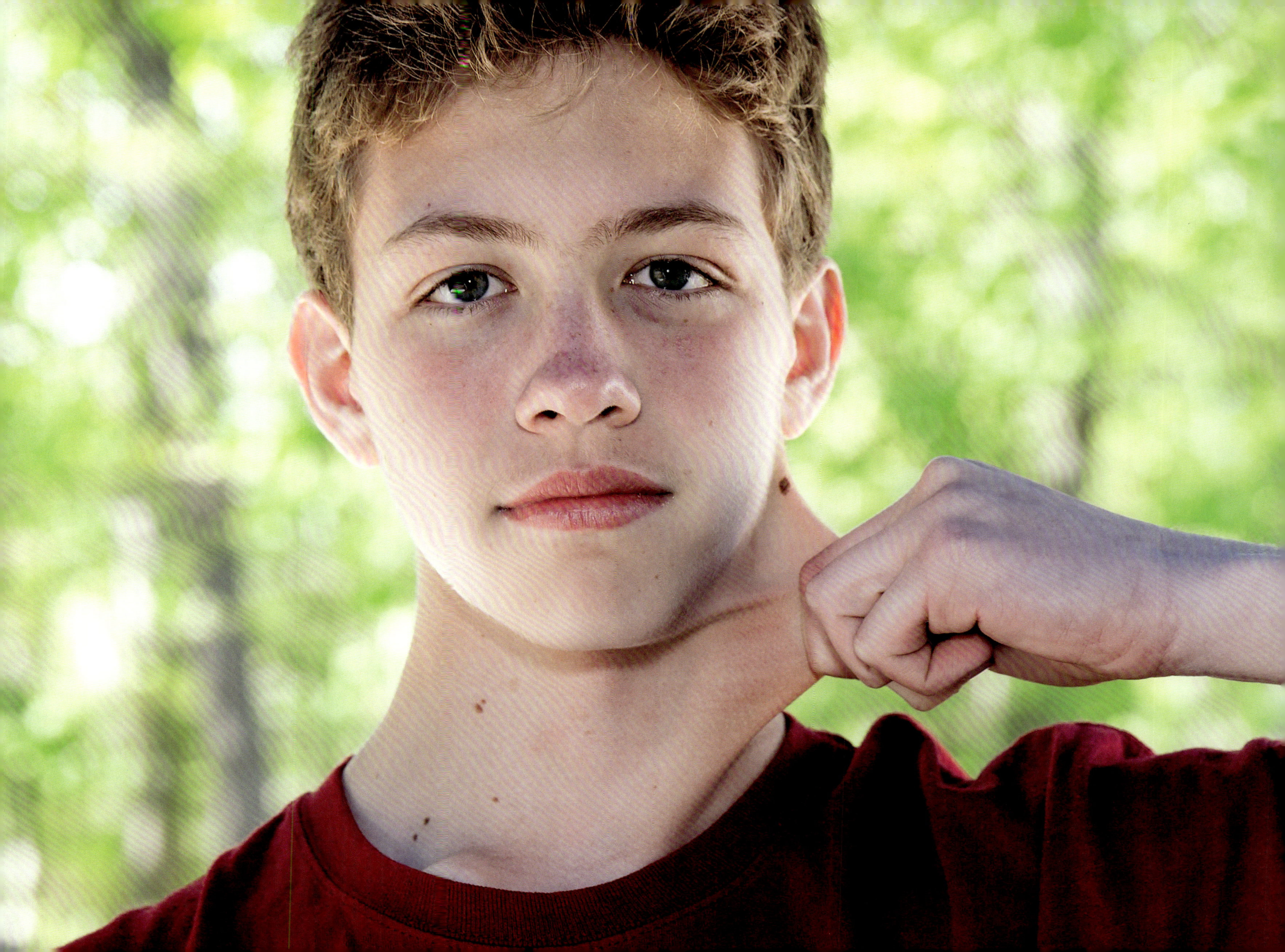

I was slightly overwhelmed. I burst into tears when I first heard because when I hear hypermobility (joints that move more than expected) I thought, "Wow. This is going to affect my life." I was crying, and instead of the doctor explaining the condition, he dismissed me and said, "Want some chocolate milk?" – Louis

It's upsetting to think about, that now people are going to look at you and say, "This kid's not normal." I have friends who can't handle what I go through so they pull away and drop me, and then there are other friends who try to give you things to make you feel better and you don't want that either. Very overwhelming. – Louis

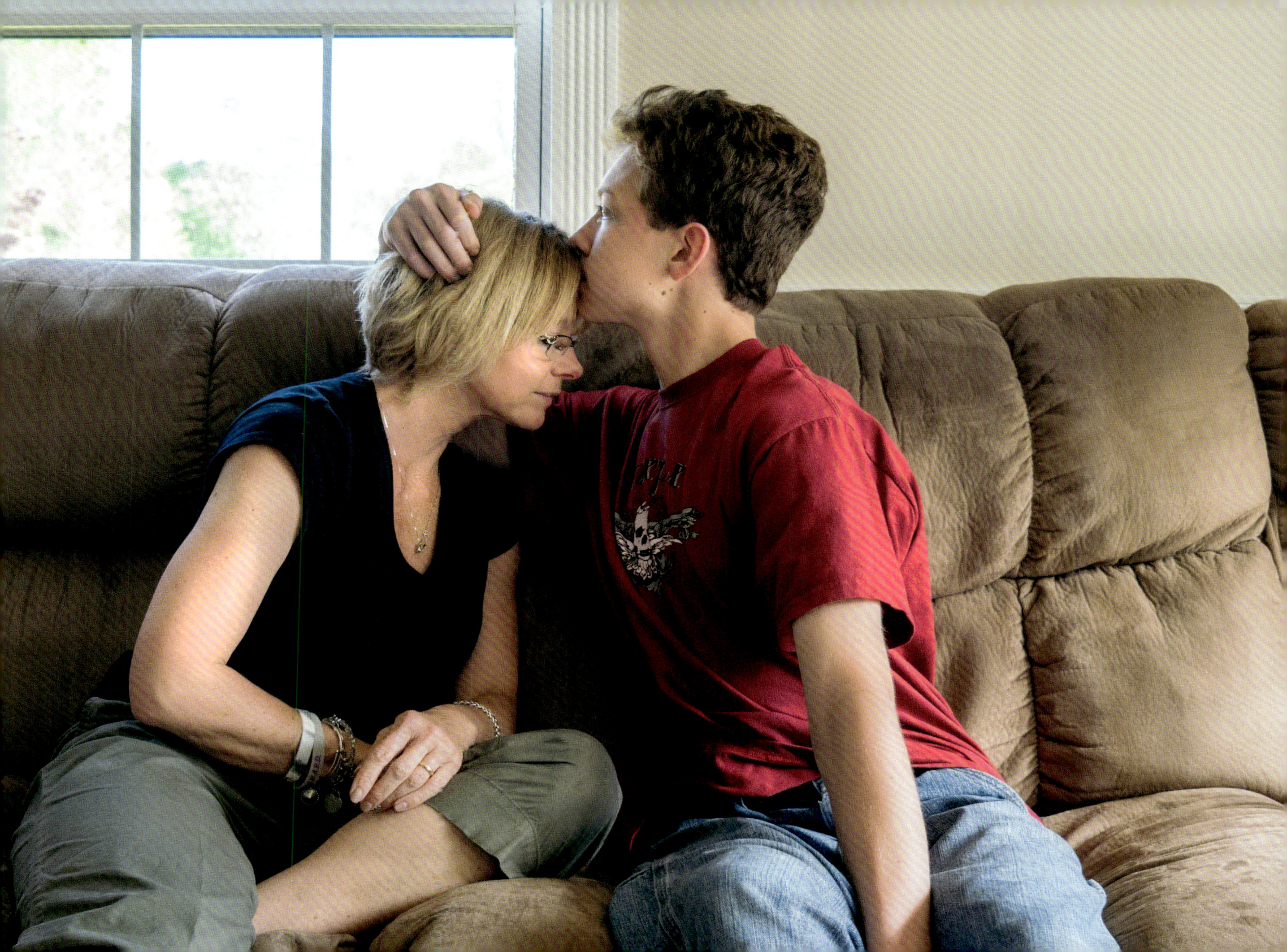

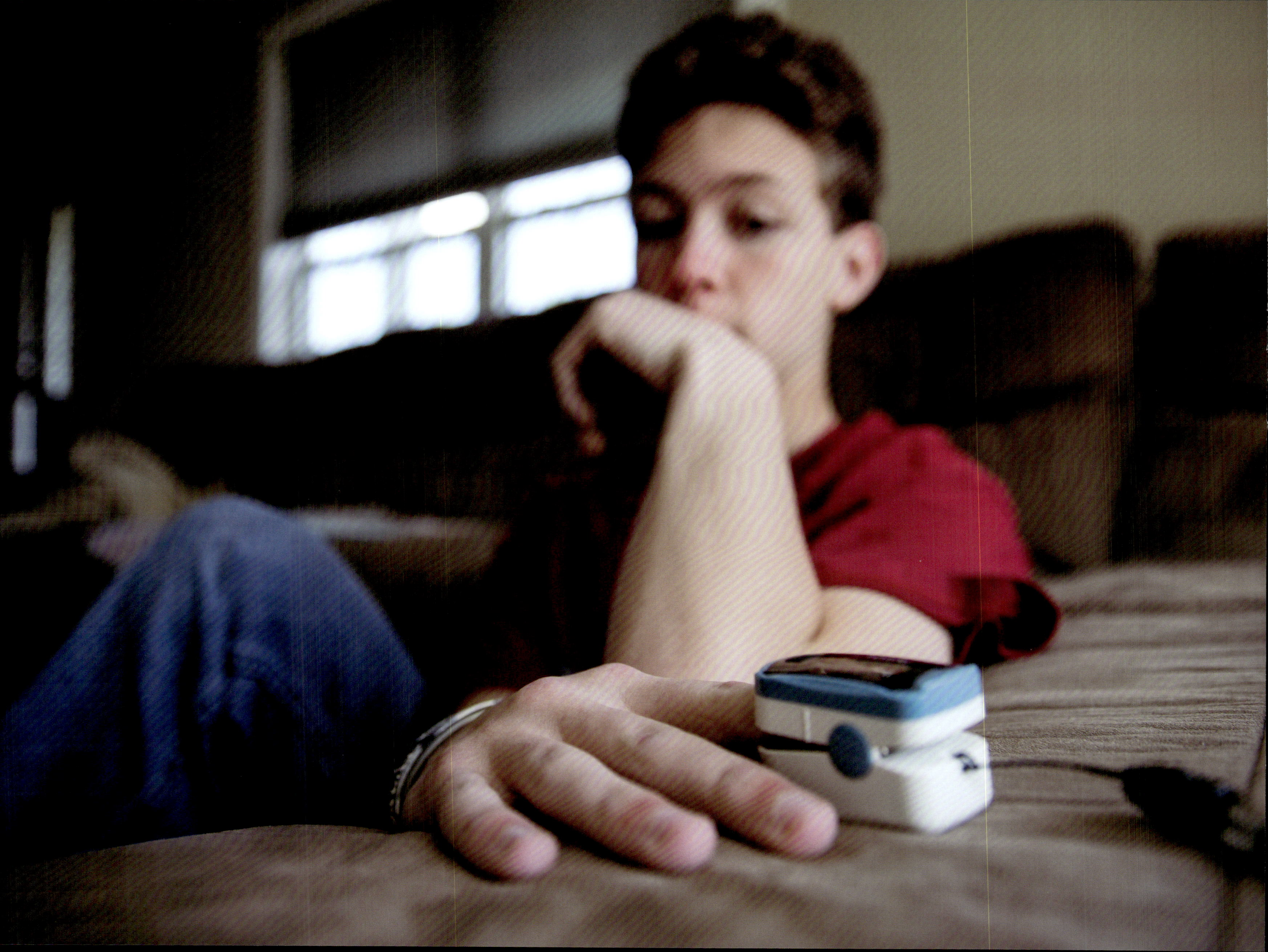

It's affected a lot of things I love. For starters, it affected my running. I used to love running until I dislocated my knee. It's affected my drumming because my shoulder can pop out so I had to stop that for a little bit. It's affected my school work because mainly after I've done so many things, my fatigue is just death.
– Louis

LOUIS'S HEART RATE OFTEN DROPS DANGEROUSLY LOW CAUSING DIZZINESS AND EXTREME FATIGUE. MONITORING IT FREQUENTLY IS CRITICAL.

I'm really afraid of just getting severely hurt. I'm afraid that I'm going to think I'm up for something, like hanging out with people, then something's going to happen and I'm just going to feel helpless and hurt. – Louis

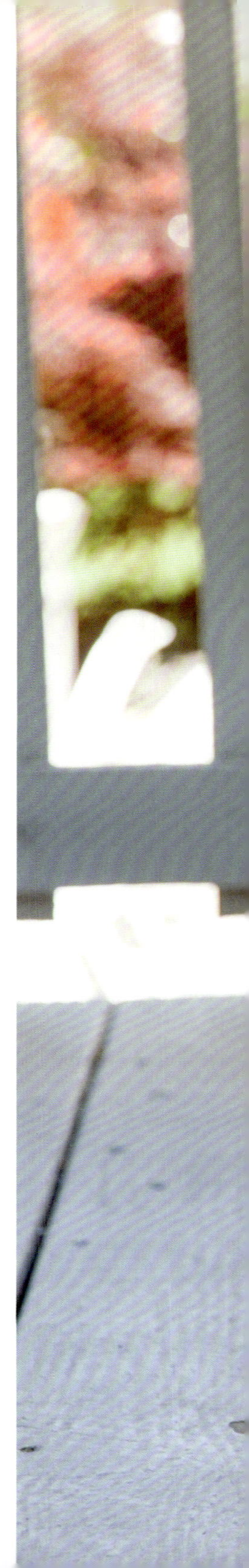

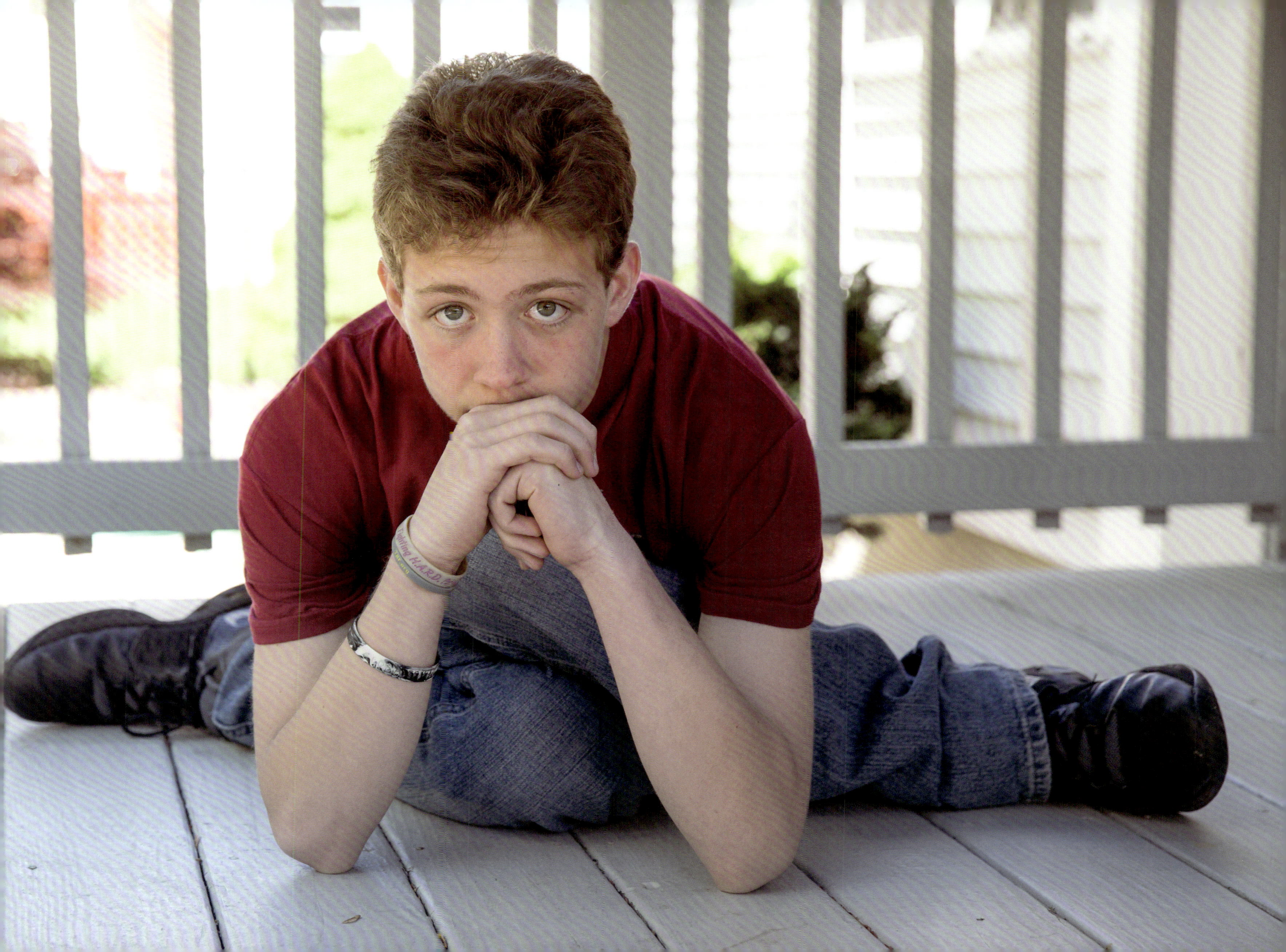

WHILE GETTING AN ULTRASOUND ON HIS NECK, JAMESY'S DAD REALIZED THAT HIS SON'S LEG SPASMS MAY IMPROVE THROUGH SIMILAR THERAPY. HE ADMINISTERS IT EVERY OTHER DAY. AFTER A FEW MONTHS, HE SAW DRAMATIC IMPROVEMENT IN JAMESY'S MOTOR FUNCTION.

Jamesy

Jamesy, 7, has Duchenne Muscular Dystrophy, a genetic disorder that weakens the muscles. Shortly after his diagnosis, his father started JAR of Hope, an organization that seeks to raise both awareness and funds for research. Jamesy is also the first duchenne patient to treat his leg pain with ultrasound therapy, an idea that occurred to his father during a routine visit to the chiropractor. Jamesy loves video games, legos, and his stuffed animal, Freddy.

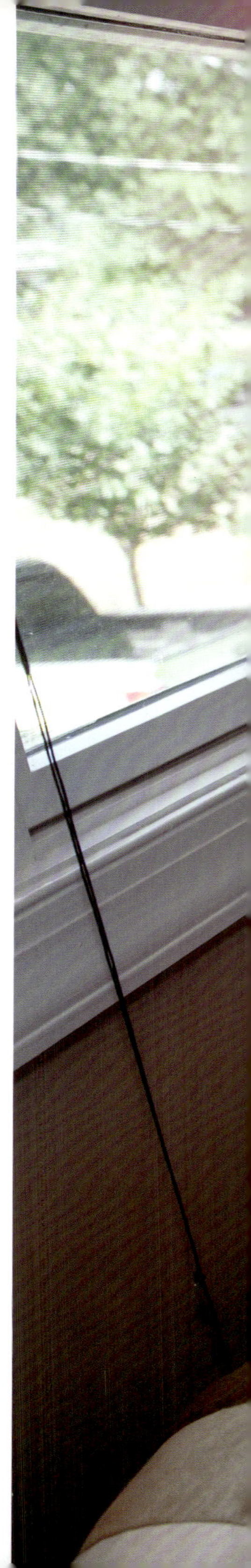

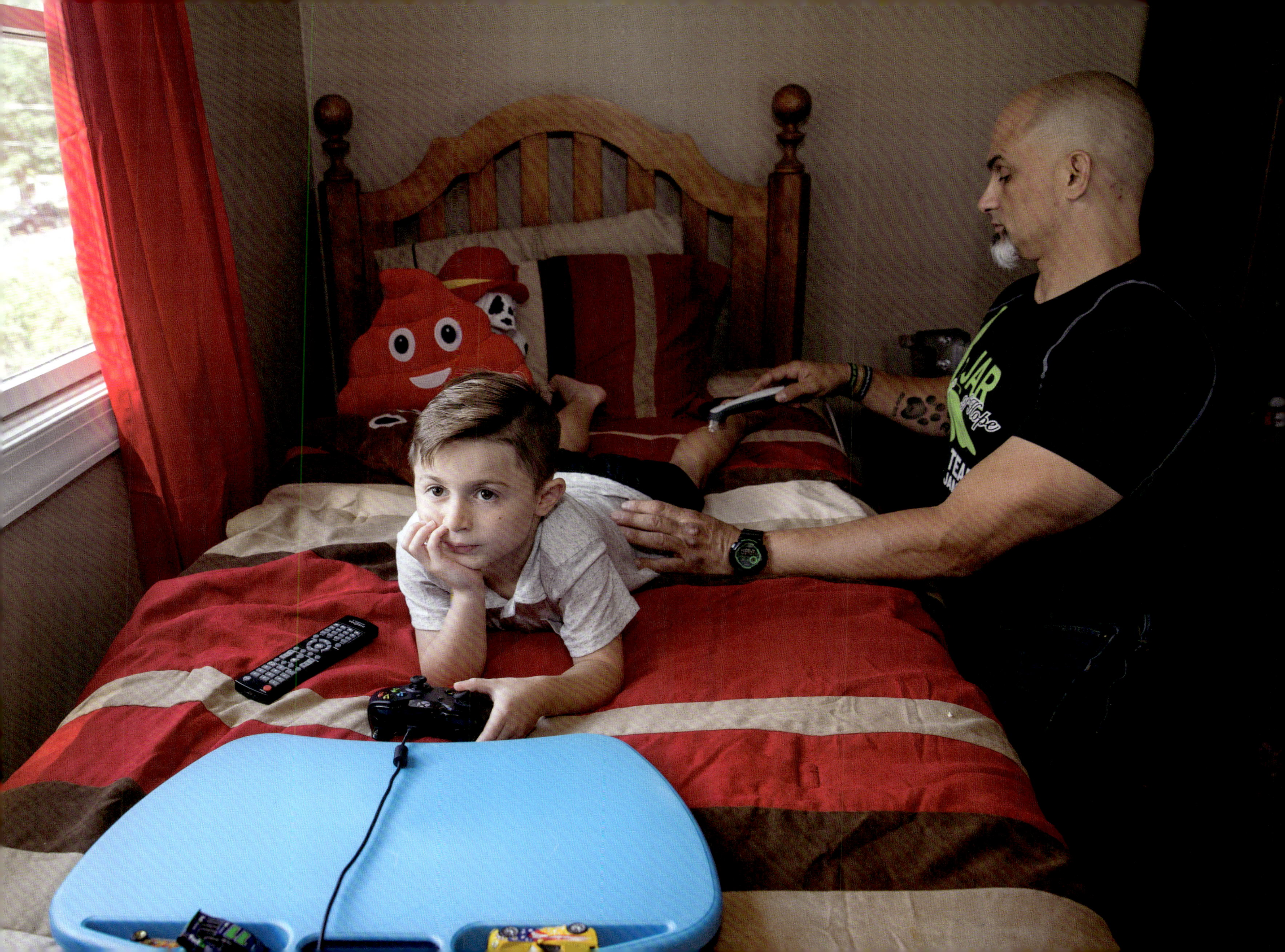

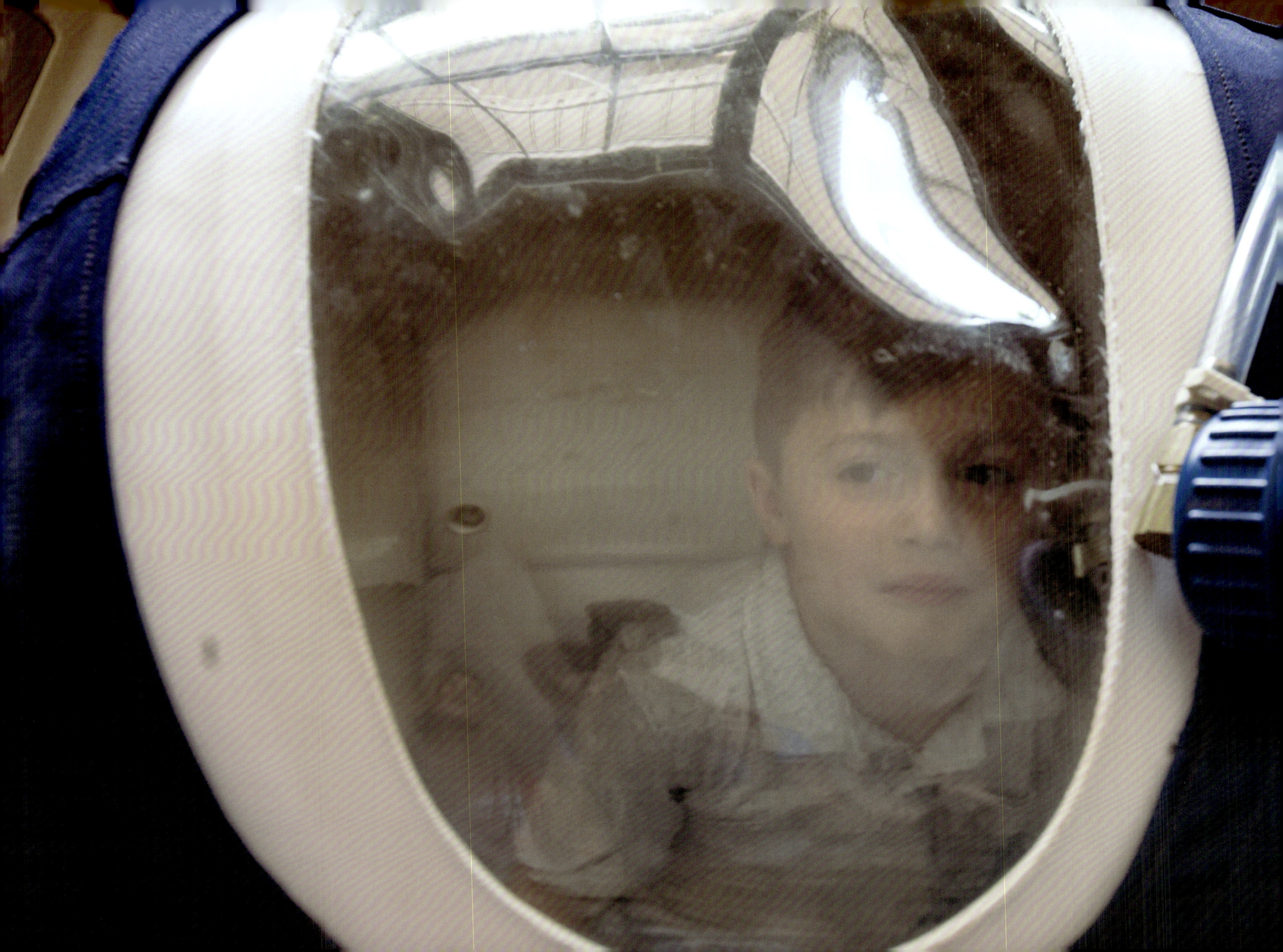

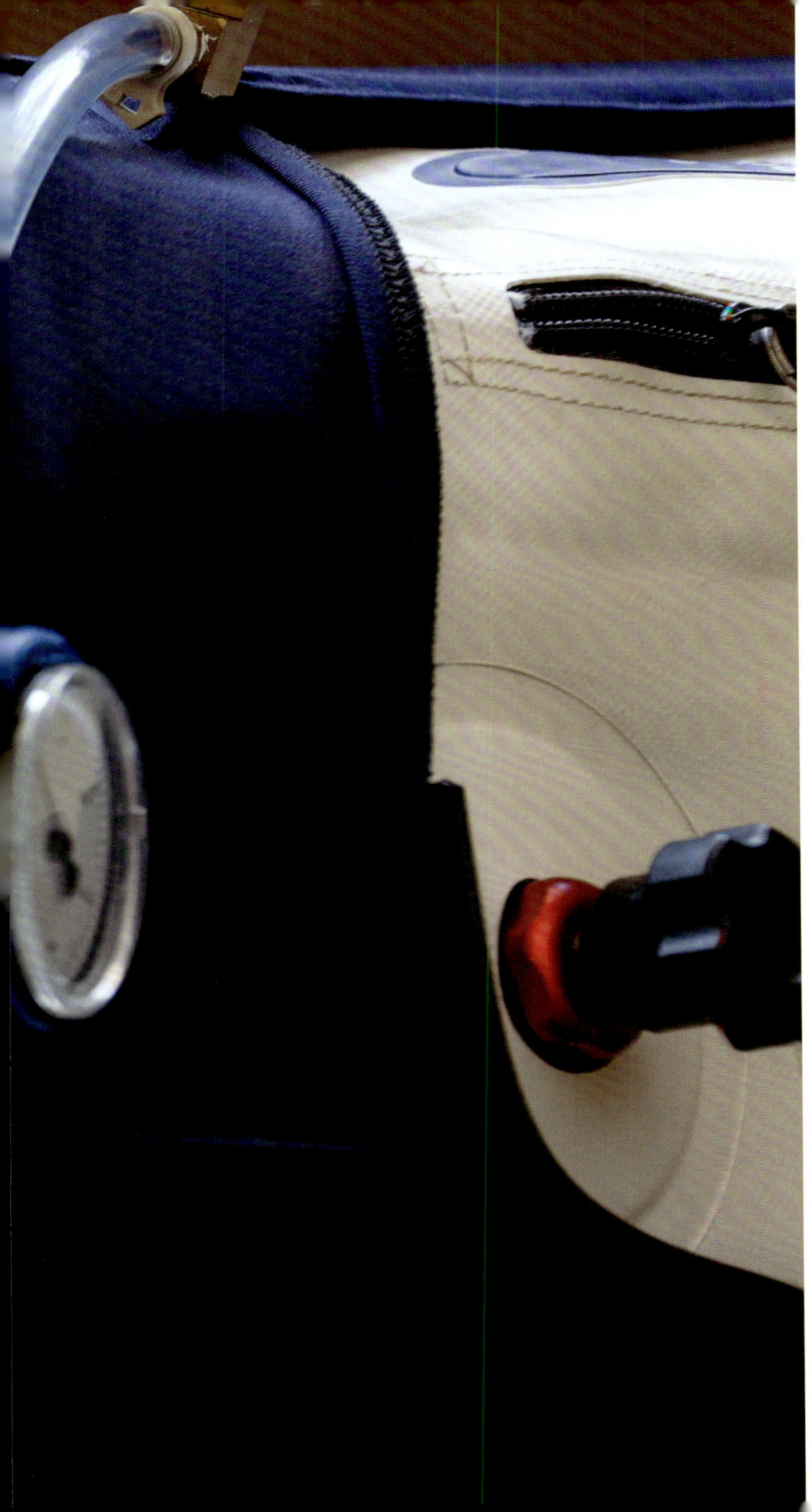

I don't know what was worse: hearing what he was sick with or the fact that she reiterated time and time again there is nothing we can do for him. You're expecting okay he is sick, this is the protocol, this is what we are going to do. Not even surgery, not even chemo, not even the strongest steroids. There is just nothing. Go home and love your son.
– Jim, Jamesy's father

I said, "Doc, you've got to listen to me, I got to explain to you what's going on with my son." And after a couple of hours he said, "Alright, I don't know you, let me talk to someone you know." I gave him some references and lo and behold the next day he called me back and said, "I have the machine for you. Take it home and try to save your son's life."
– Jim, Jamesy's father

JAMESY'S FATHER, AFTER HEARING OF THE POTENTIAL BENEFIT OF A HYPERBARIC CHAMBER IN A SEMINAR, SECURED A MACHINE TO TEST IT WITH HIS SON. JAMESY'S CARDIAC AND PULMONARY FUNCTIONS IMPROVED. JAR OF HOPE AND THE UNIVERSITY OF MINN. ARE PARTNERING TO CONDUCT FURTHER RESEARCH INTO THIS TREATMENT.

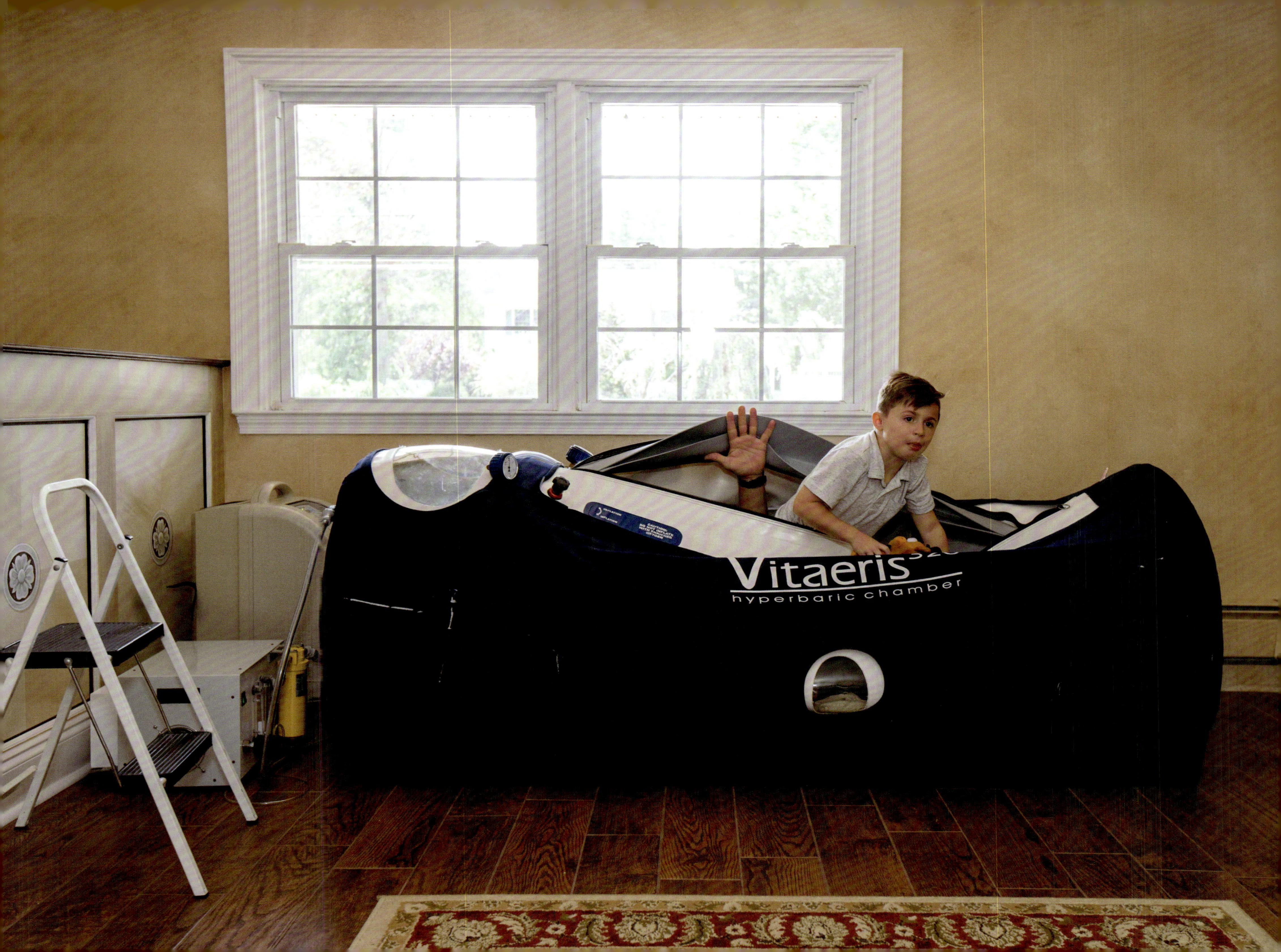
Vitaeris
hyperbaric chamber

The most important statistic for me is my son, by the age of 9 to 12 can end up in a wheelchair. He'll lose his ability to walk, and if that happens, the science community says that no matter what drugs come out, they won't try them on these kids because their bodies are to ravaged with scar tissue, and too tough to reverse it. So not only is his body going to break down in a very demeaning way, but the sands are literally seeping through the hourglass.
– Jim, Jamesy's father

JAMESY GETS UPSET ON THE NIGHTS THAT HE SPENDS INSIDE THE CHAMBER SO HIS FATHER SLEEPS NEXT TO HIM.

We had—for complete transparency—talked about clearing the garage out and putting the family in a car and turning the car on and just all going together. – Jim, Jamesy's father

I'll never forget it, [Jim] said, "I gave you the weekend, that's it, now we're gonna fight." And I said, "I can't, I can't. I lost my father when I was 13, I lost my mother when I was 30, I don't have fight in me." He said, "Well just follow me." And even today that's all I do, is I follow him, whatever he tells me that's what I do. – Karen, Jamesy's mother

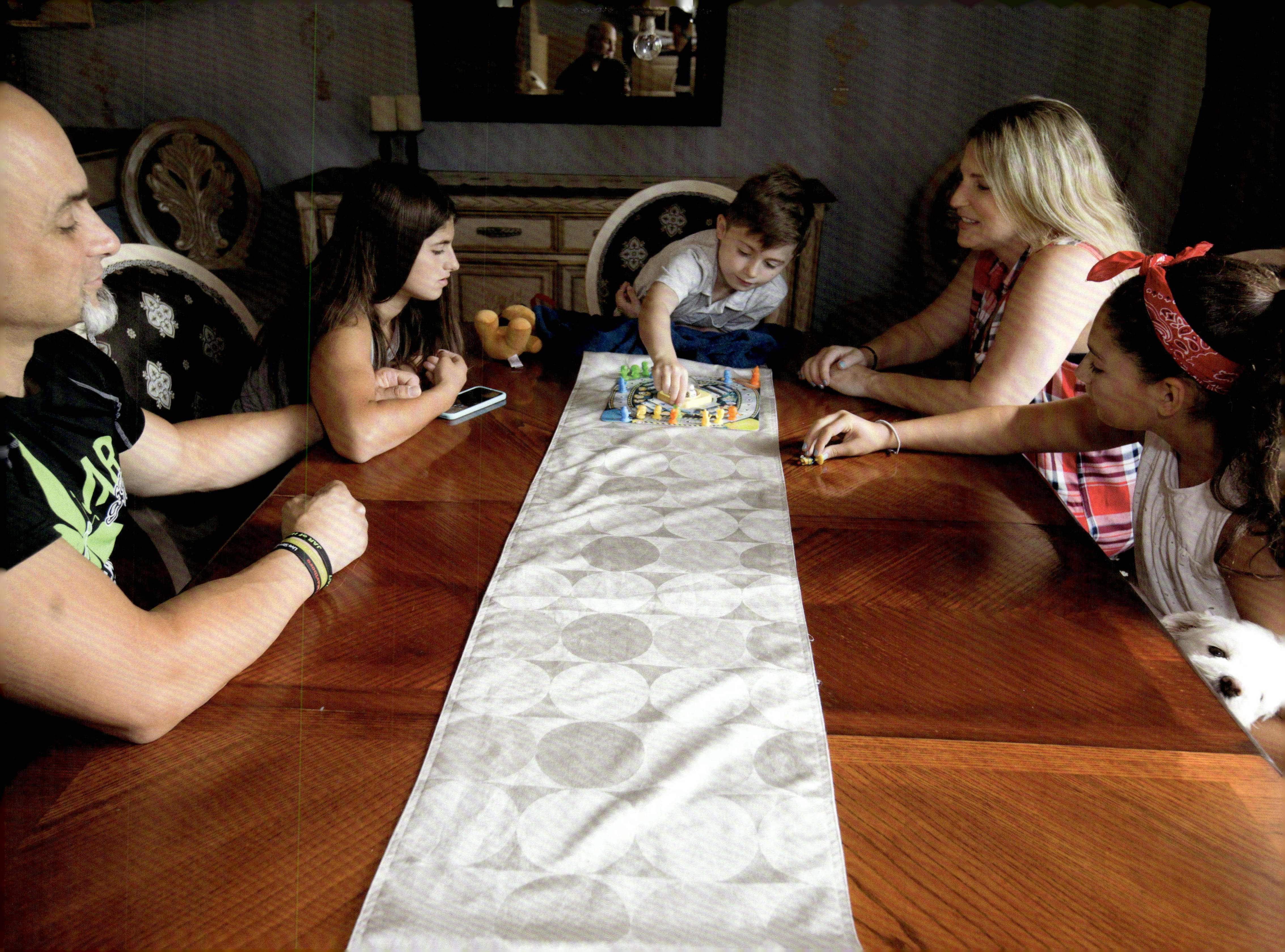

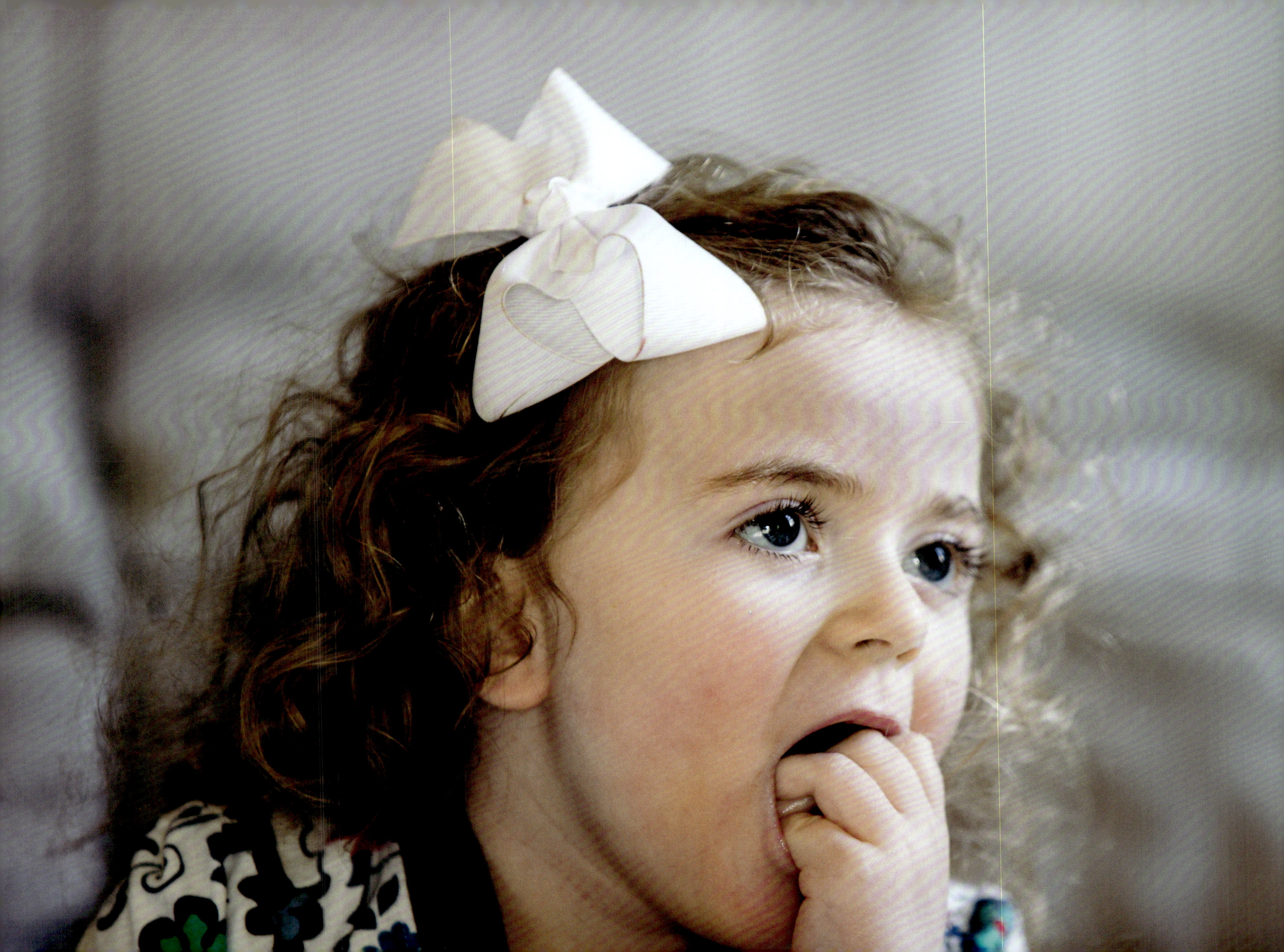

People don't get it unless they live it. I might be at Taryn's school when a mom might be like, "How's Brynn? Is she walking yet?" "No, she's not walking." "Oh, I feel so bad for you." I'm sitting in the middle of the cafeteria at school. I'm like, "Oh, it's okay, thanks." It's almost like you want to just not go there and have a conversation. – Kristen, Brynn's mother

She used to crawl and now she doesn't, so that was devastating. Then, when they mentioned G-tube (feeding tube), that was super scary for me. In hindsight, we have to keep her healthy and it put pounds on her and it's working. We've had no issues so we're happy with our decision, but that's our job, to keep Brynn healthy and strong until, ultimately, there's a treatment for her. That's our hope. – Kristen, Brynn's mother

Brynn

Brynn's development seemed relatively normal to her parents until, at 9 months old, she still showed no signs of crawling. At the age of two, a blood test determined that Brynn had Rett syndrome, a neurological disorder most common in girls. Though most children with Rett initially develop at a normal pace, they eventually lose use of their hands, experience delayed brain and head growth, have difficulty walking, suffer from seizures, and are intellectually disabled. Brynn, 5, is not able to walk or talk, but she loves music, horseback riding, and being read to.

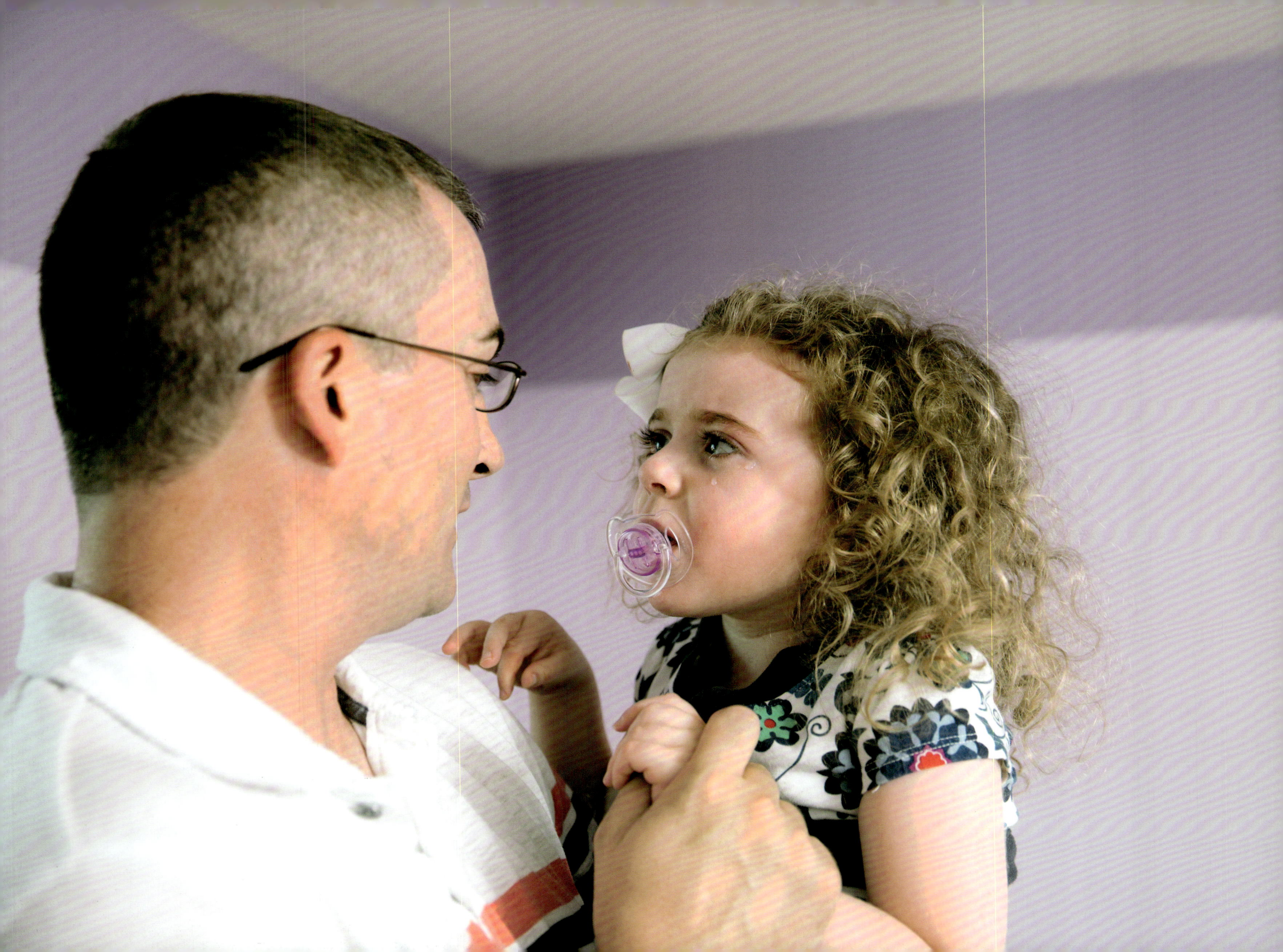

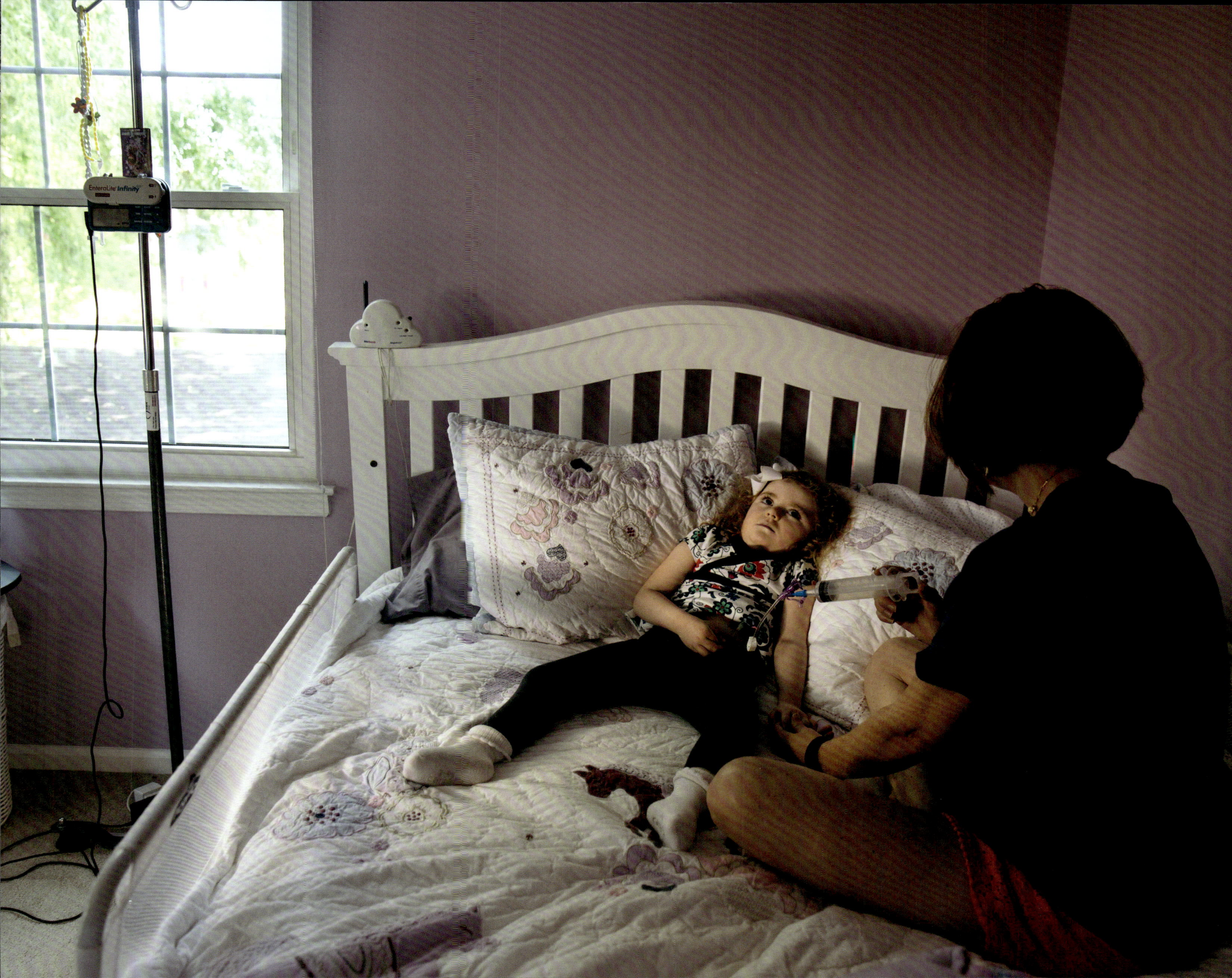
EnteraLite Infinity

Unless my son is yellowish, with bags under his eyes, or has petechiae, which are the dots on his body, you would look at my child and say, "You have a healthy child," and you would think they were crazy, and they're not crazy because the blood tests don't lie.
– Karen, Nico's mother

Cutest thing ever is he actually was able to go inside McDonald's for the first time and he says, "I didn't know you could go inside!" He came home with his sister and he said, "Mom, guess what? You can go in, too!" We take nothing for granted. Nothing. – Karen, Nico's mother

Nico

Though Nico, 4, often appears to be in perfect health, he is one of less than 1,000 children around the world suffering from Evans syndrome, Idiopathic thrombocytopenic purpura, and Neutropenia, an autoimmune disorder. Sickness as mild as a common cold frequently escalates, requiring Nico to be hospitalized. Because his immune system is so weak, Nico is not able to be in many public places, including school. Evans syndrome is not heavily researched and the cause is still unknown. Nico loves toys, arts and crafts, baking, the outdoors, and dreams of owning a zoo one day. His latest interest has been science, as he wants to make medicine for sick people.

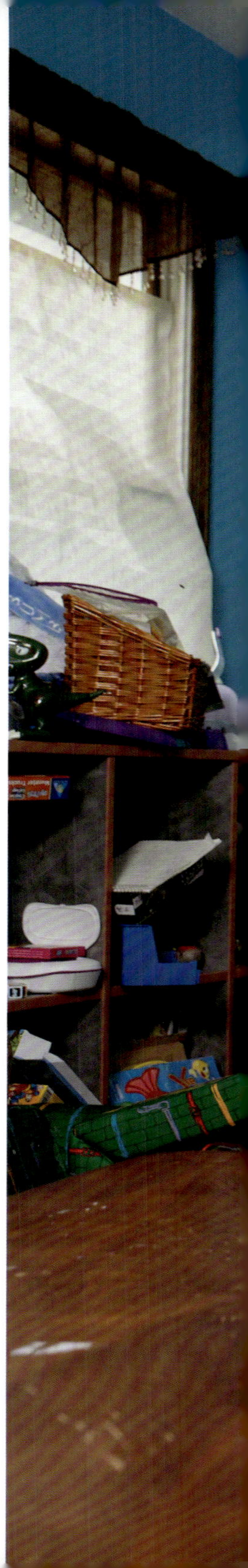

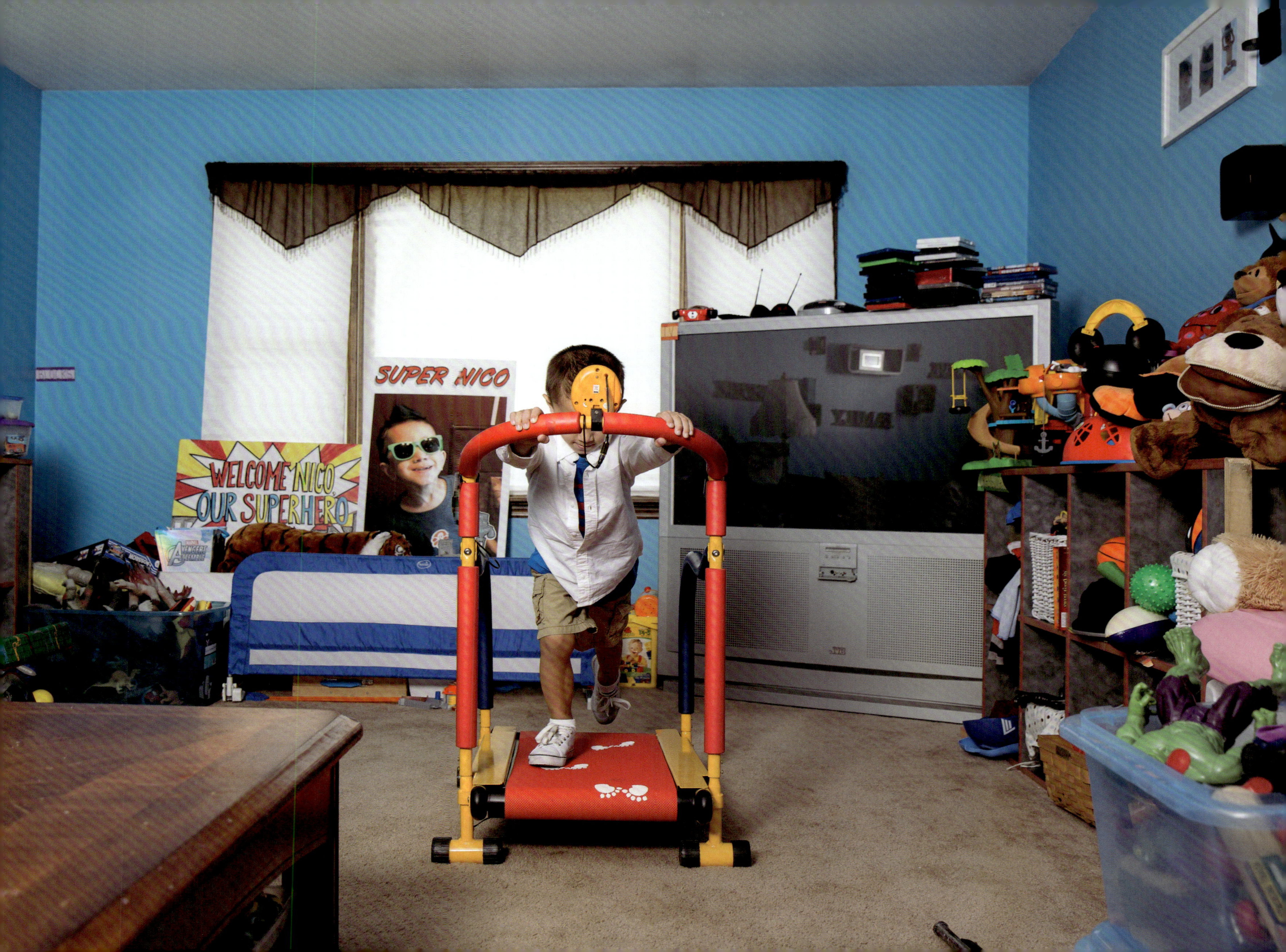

SUPER NICO
WELCOME NICO OUR SUPERHERO

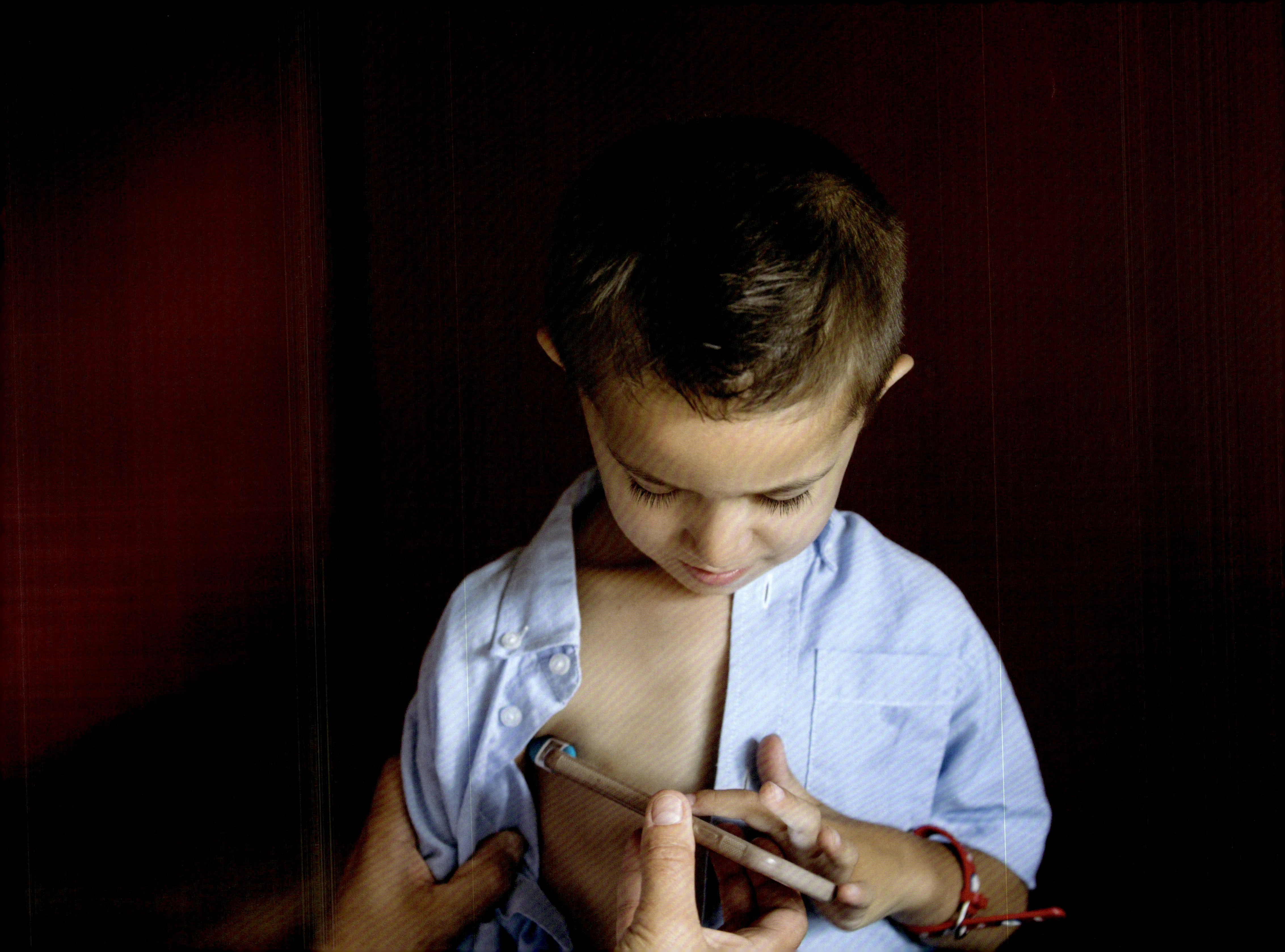

Our biggest challenge is outside assistance for our family. Because he doesn't have cancer, but he's treated at the Cancer Institute, it's almost like we're on the outside, looking in.
– Karen, Nico's mother

NICO'S TEMPERATURE IS MONITORED WITH AN IPHONE APP THAT ALLOWS HIM TO PLAY A GAME SIMULTANEOUSLY.

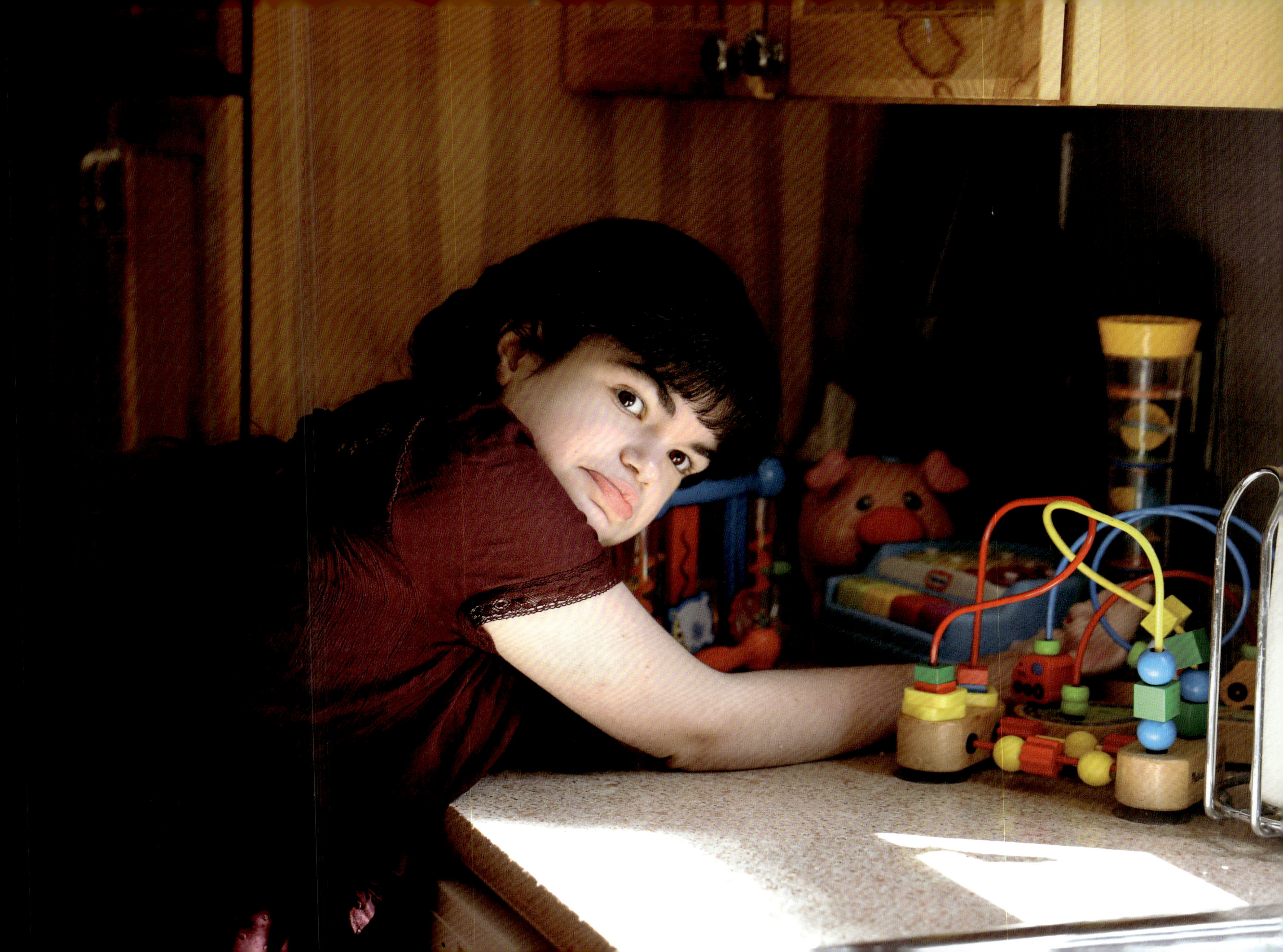

Emily has taught me lessons that I never would have had without her. I am more patient. I am kind. I have compassion like I never knew was possible. I have learned that doctors do not know everything, and know very little about ultra-rare genetic disorders. I have learned that I am a damn good voice for my daughter. I have found strength in places and situations that you'd never know strength could be found in. I have learned to take a lot of deep breaths. I have learned that it's okay to just cry sometimes. I have learned that even with all of these lessons, I am still human. – Danielle, Emily's mom

Emily

Emily's illness is similar to Alzheimer's but in children. Sanfilippo syndrome is progressive and mainly affects the brain and spinal cord. Emily, 11, was once typical then stopped gaining skills and began to decline. She is no longer verbal and has gone from being fully potty trained to using diapers. She cannot feed or dress herself. She is considered to be around 9 months neurologically. Soon Emily will lose the ability to walk, eat, and swallow, and will end up on a feeding tube and spending her days in a chair or bed unable to move or communicate. Emily's life will end either before, or in her very early teens. There are absolutely no treatments for Sanfilippo syndrome, and that means no cure. Emily enjoys watching *iCarly*, *Drake and Josh*, and *SpongeBob*; going for walks; and visiting with others.

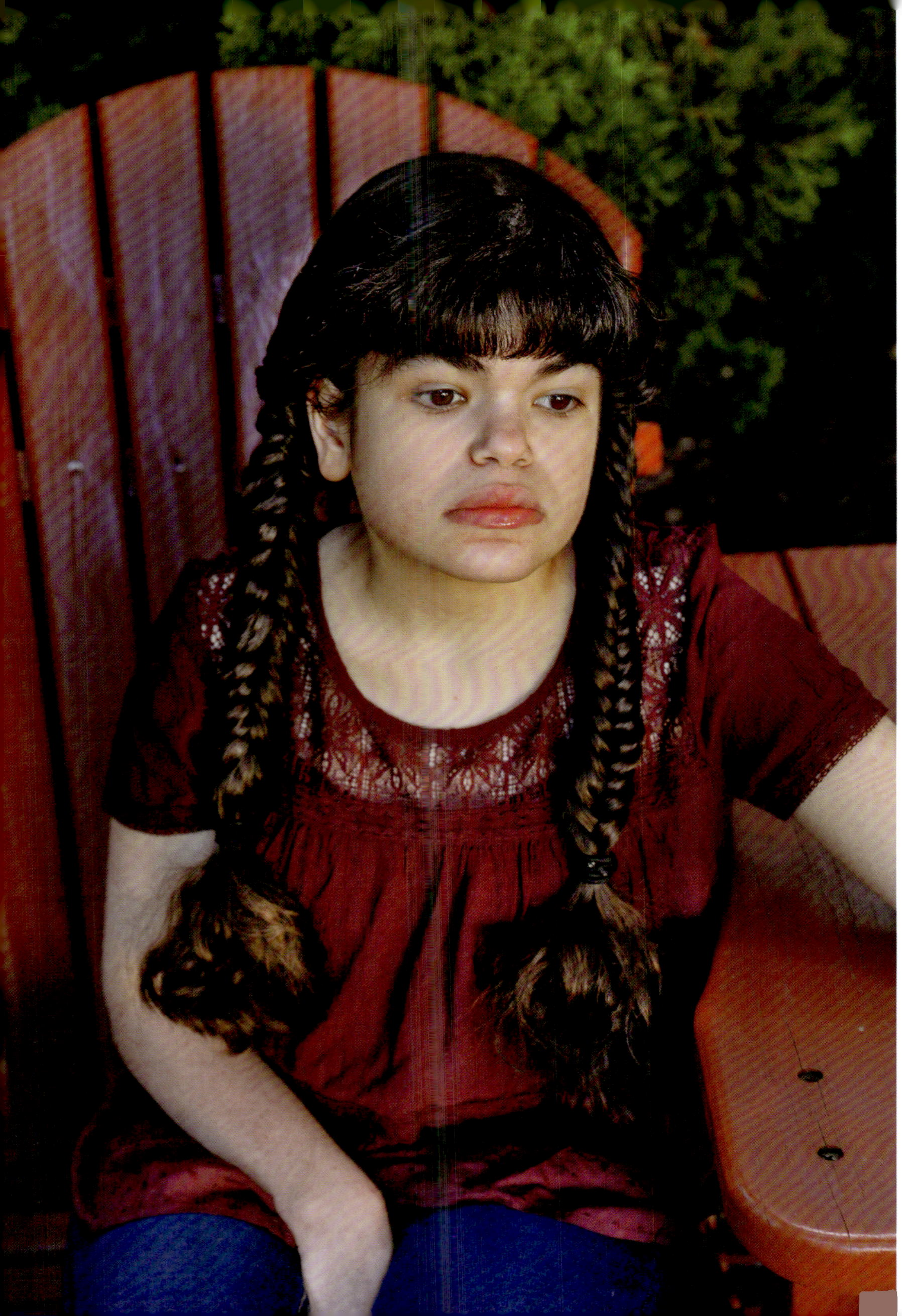

There is no such thing as just sitting back with feet up relaxing. Emily needs to be walked a lot during the night to keep her joints and everything working properly and she requires full assistance. She must never be left alone. This means that even using the bathroom with Emily home takes some planning. There are no vacations since most money is spent on supplements and Emily's needs. As a caregiver, my physical being is very negatively affected. I have gained 100 pounds since her diagnosis. – Danielle, Emily's mom

My future fear, and there is only one, is Emily's death. – Danielle, Emily's mom

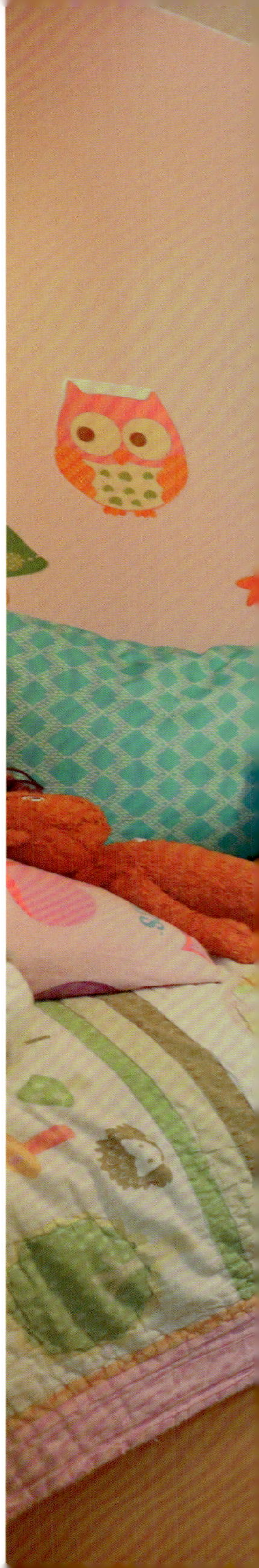

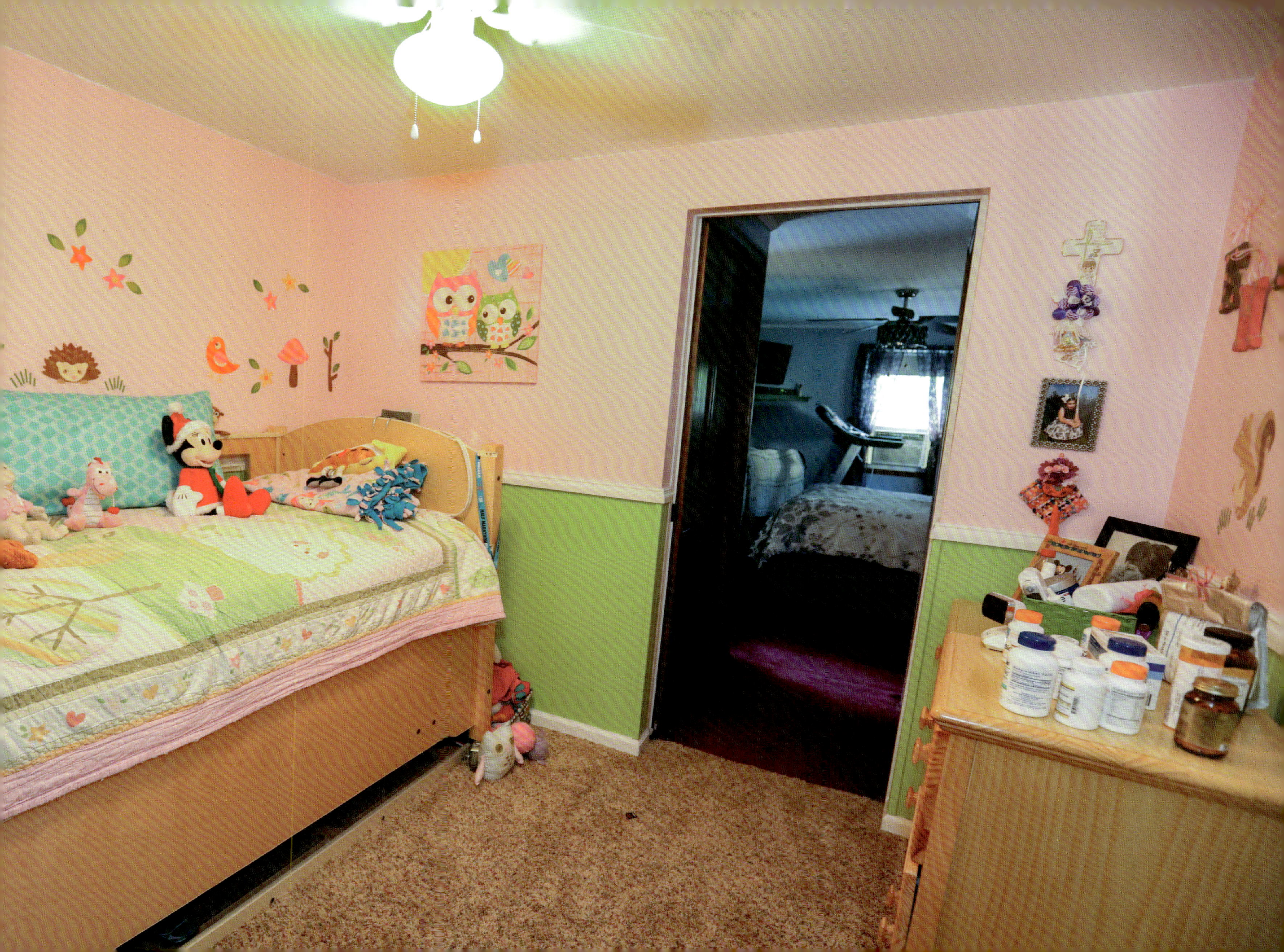

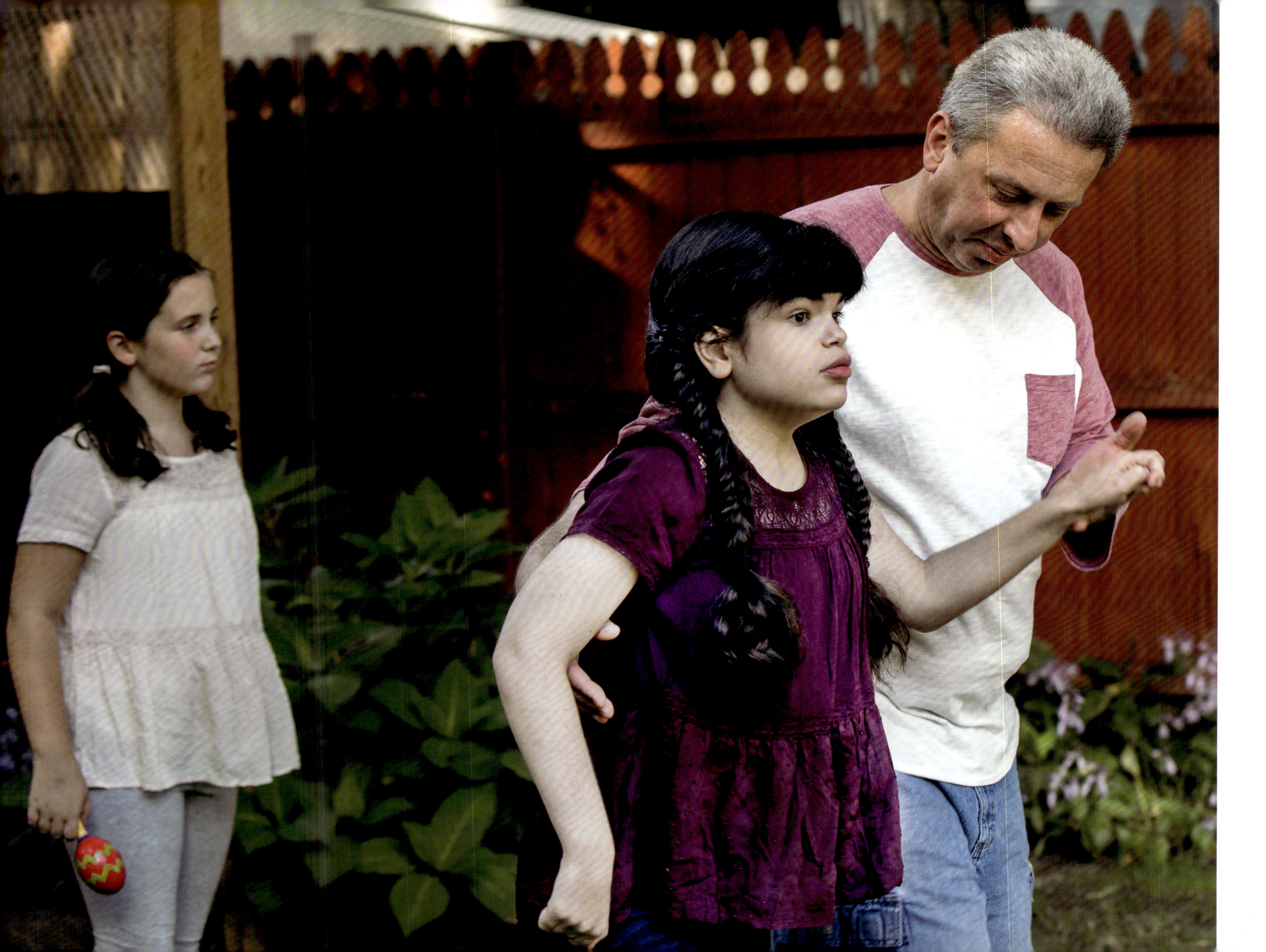

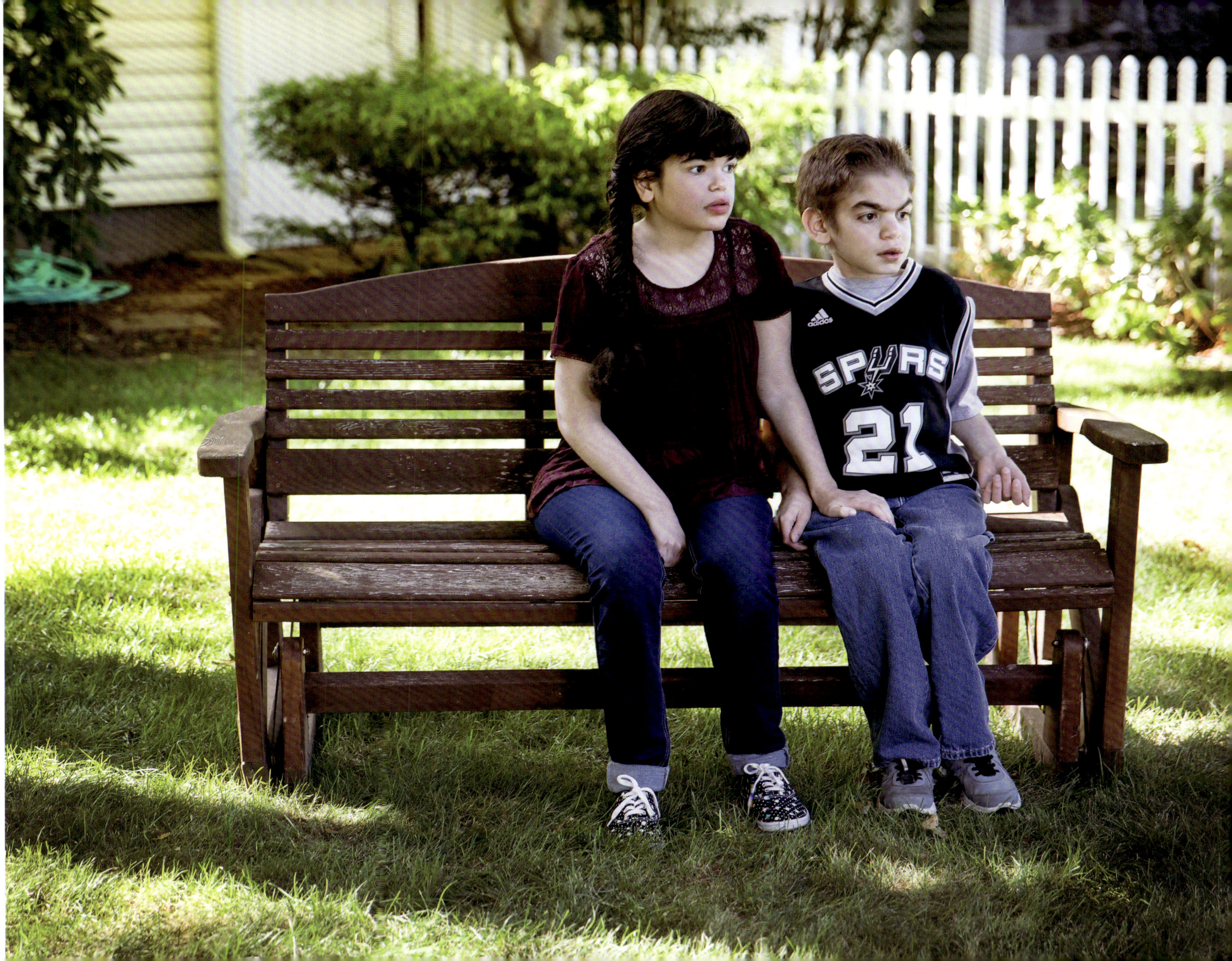
adidas
SPURS
21

I think that the more I'm researching about genetic disorders and the more people I'm coming into contact with, I may be realizing that it's maybe more than meets the eye, and maybe I can stop blaming myself. – Eliza, Daniel's mother

Daniel

Though Daniel's parents first noticed developmental issues at 9 months, they did not receive his diagnosis, Glass syndrome, until about two years ago. At 5, Daniel has trouble with his fine and gross motor skills and is nonverbal. There is still very little known about this disorder. Daniel loves playing with cars, especially ones that have doors that open and close. He also loves bubbles and bringing his suitcase around.

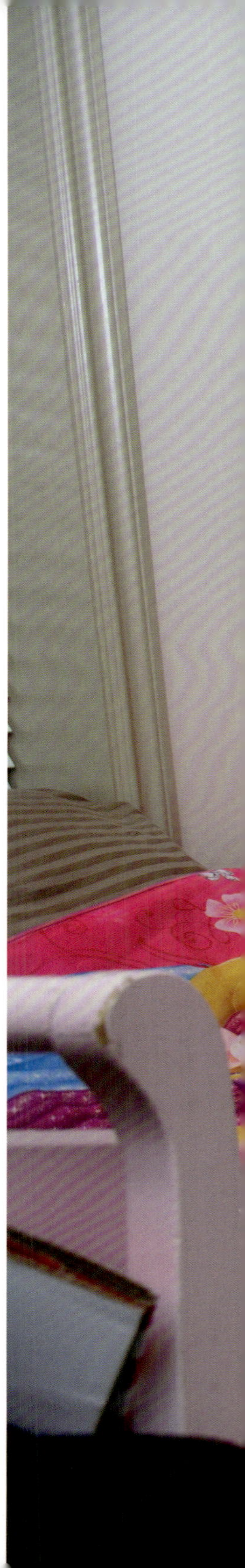

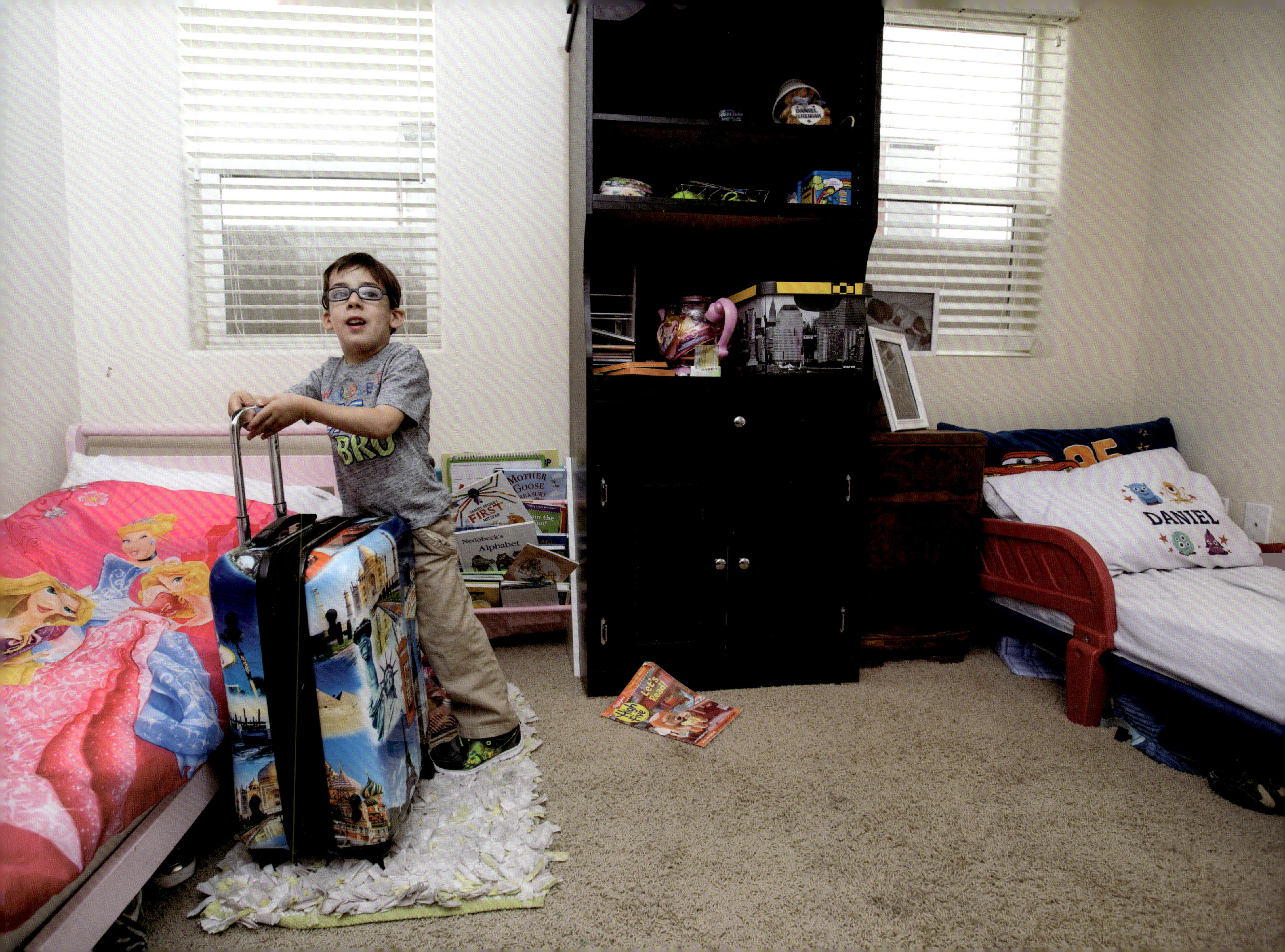
BRO
MOTHER GOOSE TREASURY
FIRST
Nedobeck's Alphabet
Let's Read!
DANIEL

Brian's cognition will always stay intact, he'll always be smart, and he'll always know what's going on, but his body systems will deteriorate and/or fail as he gets older. So we've decided that every day we're going to try to make it special, and every day we're going to try to watch him laugh, and every day we're going to just try to make the most of what we have because we don't know what the timeline is. – Lauren, Brian's mother

Brian

As a toddler, Brian, 5, never came out of the "drunken sailor" phase. At three years old, Brian was diagnosed with Ataxia-telangiectasia, a genetic disorder that causes a multisystem disease. A-T combines symptoms of muscular dystrophy, cerebral palsy, immune deficiencies, and oftentimes cancers. Children with this condition experience problems with balance and coordination, often requiring a wheelchair by adolescence. A-T patients also face a greater risk of developing leukemia and lymphoma. With full, if not advanced, cognitive development, Brian is currently unaware of his condition. Brian is a happy, inquisitive kid who loves superheroes, especially Batman.

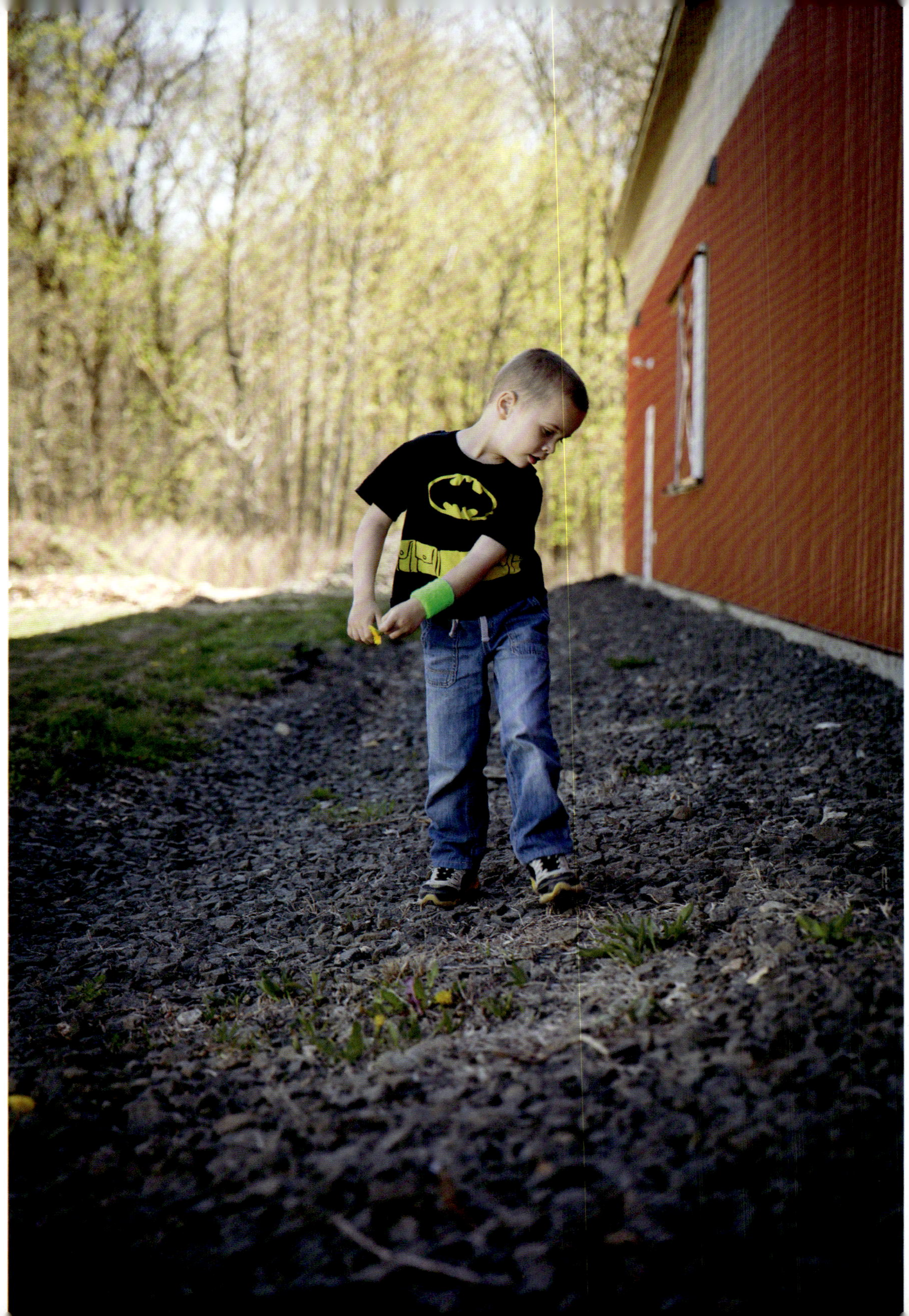

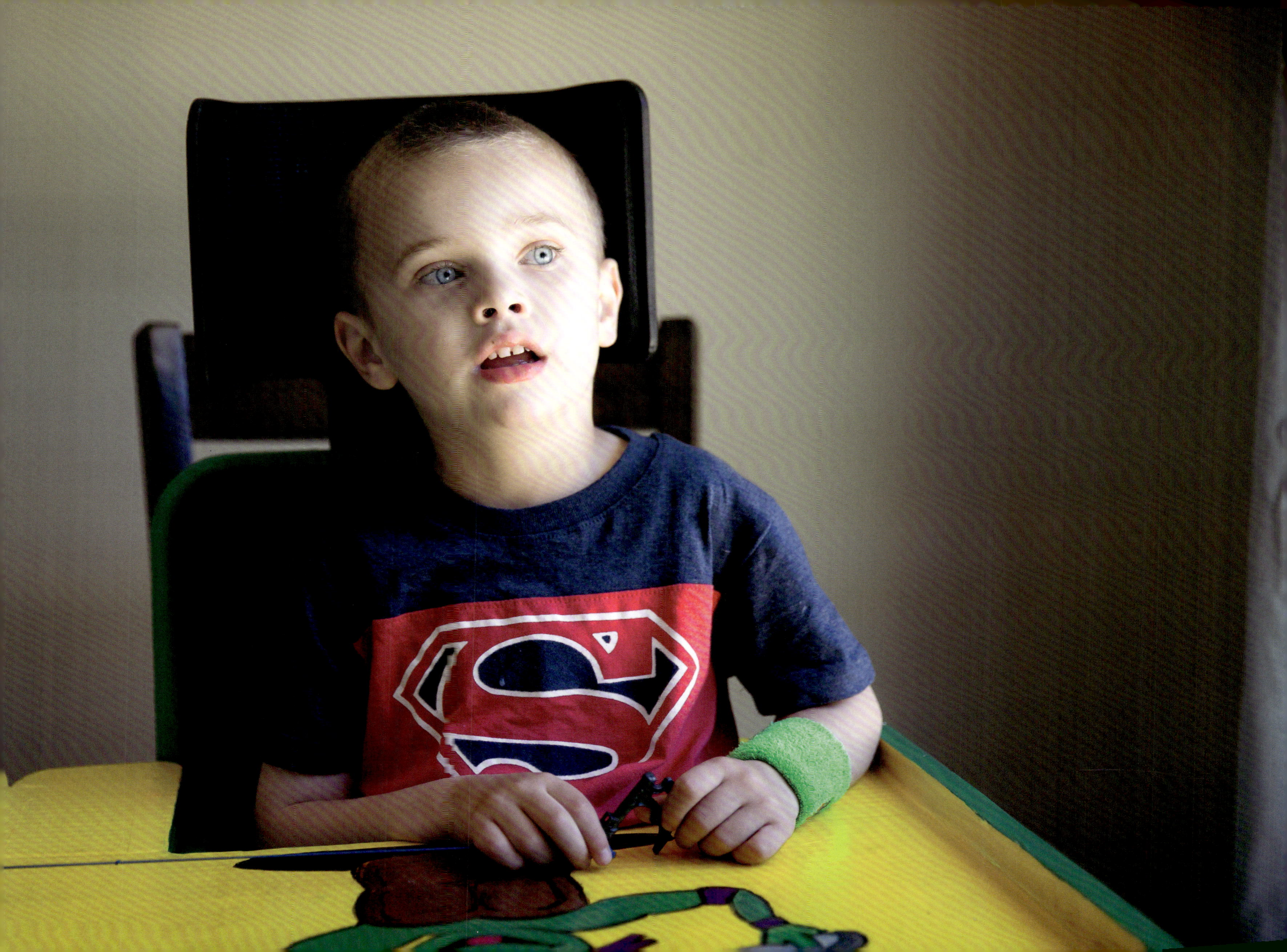

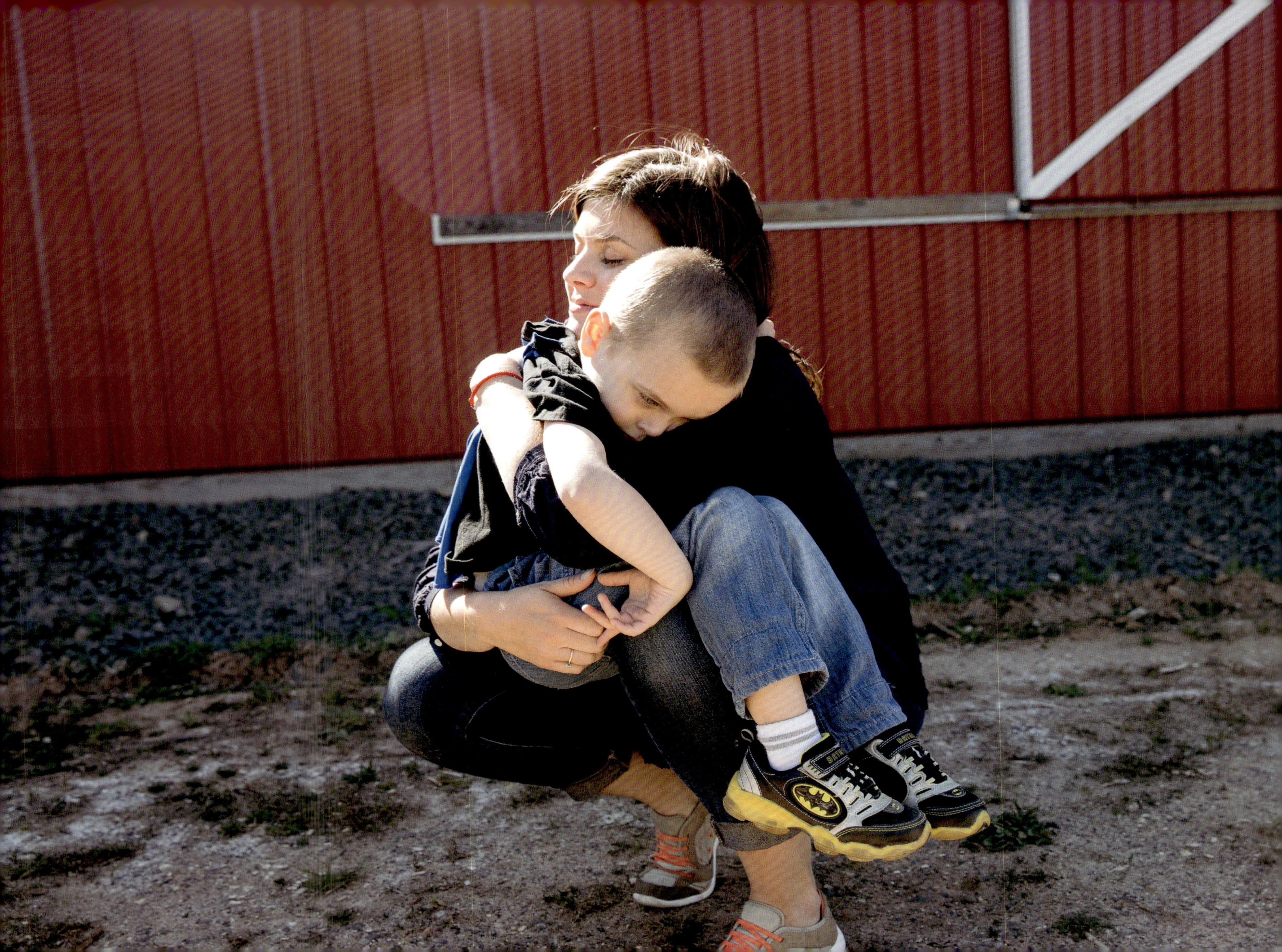

I just dread the day that we have to have the conversation with him. But there's going to come a point where the equipment is making life easier, but is also making him so very different, and at that point we will have to have the hardest conversation of our lives. We want him to be carefree as long as possible. – Lauren, Brian's mother

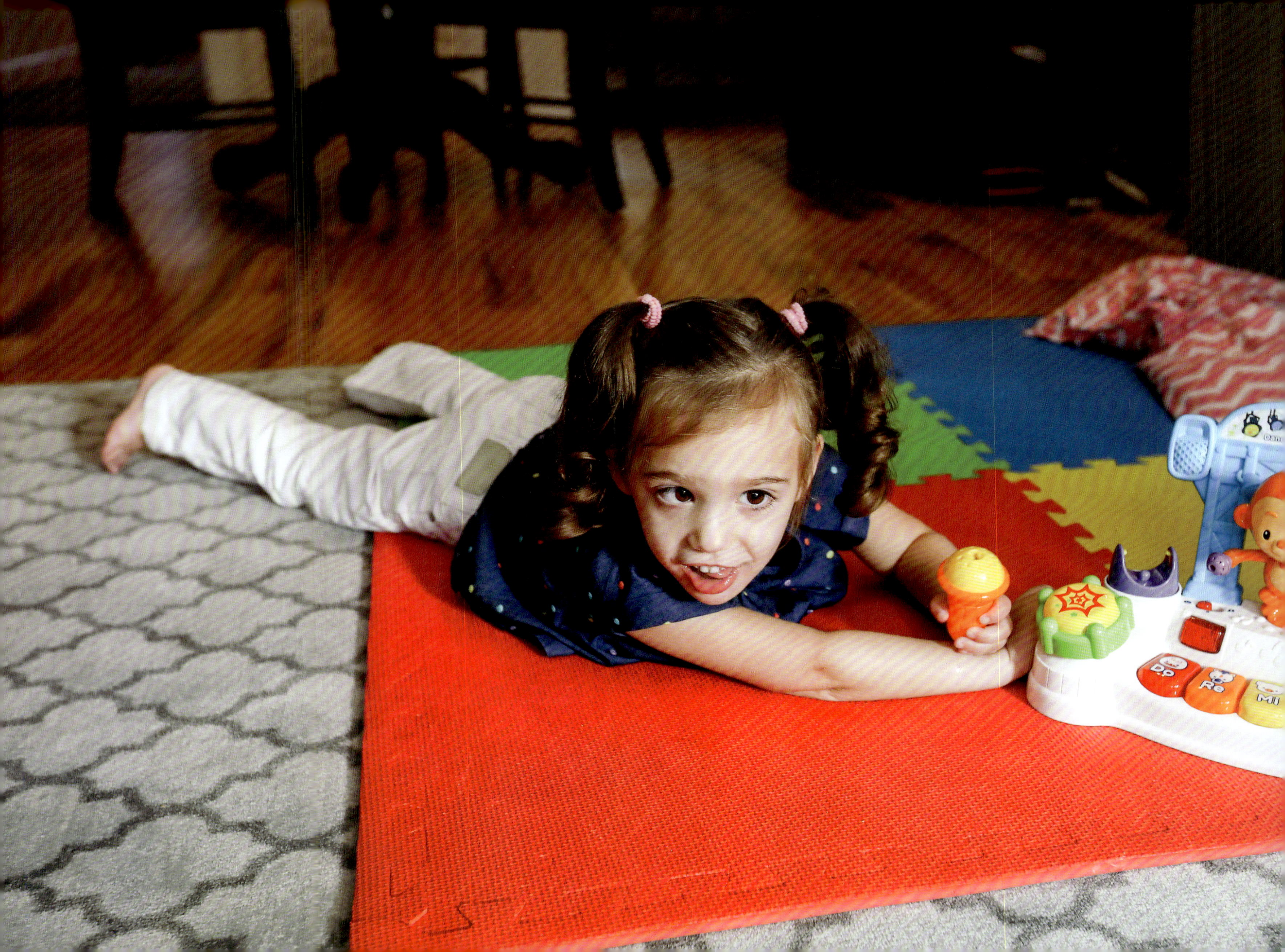
Do
Re
Mi

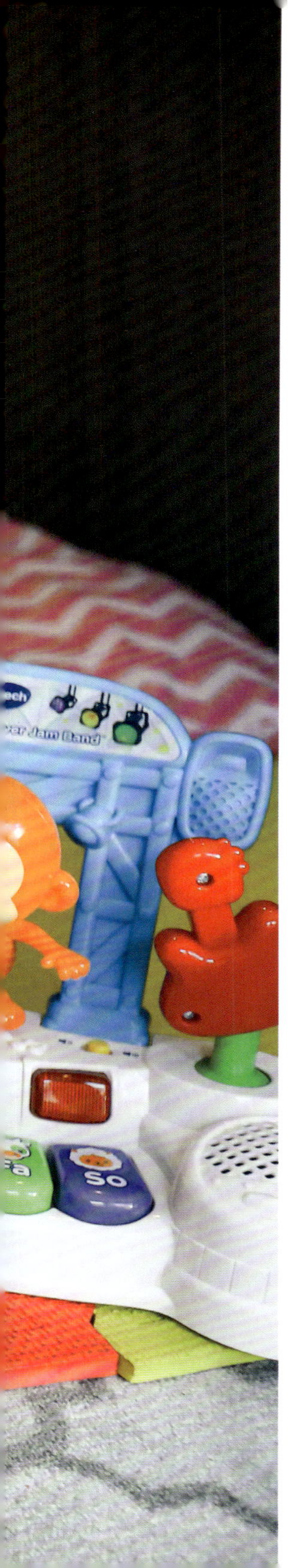

I always say this is going to be Josie's story to tell one day, because nobody can tell me that it won't be. Who knows?
– Nicole, Josie's mother

Josie

When Josie, 4, was diagnosed with FOXG1 in 2014, there were 60 people in the world known to have the neurological disorder. Almost every child with FOXG1 has a different variation of the mutation, making Josie's prognosis especially difficult. She cannot sit up unassisted. She can't talk, nor can she take care of her most basic needs. Josie has special chairs to hold her up, a gait trainer, a stander, a bath chair, a special needs stroller, and will soon have a wheelchair. Josie laughs all the time and loves playing with toys and swimming.

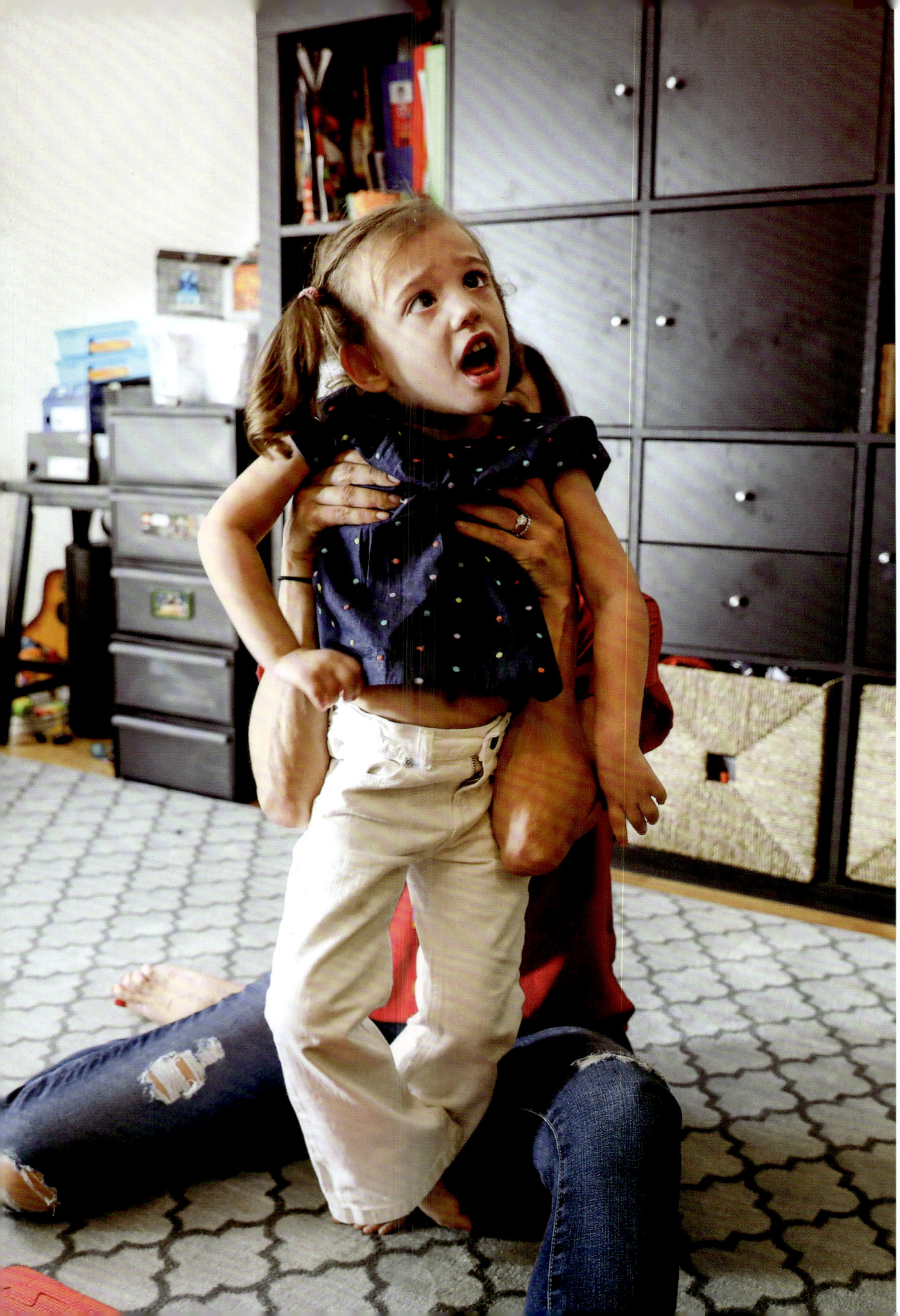

Before we had nurse care there were six months from when her seizures started till our nurse care started, that we stayed up every night. We really didn't sleep for six months. It's funny what you can do when you have to. – Nicole, Josie's mother

If you'd asked me two years ago, "Will you put Josie on a school bus?" I'd say, "no way." Things are only getting better. – Nicole, Josie's mother

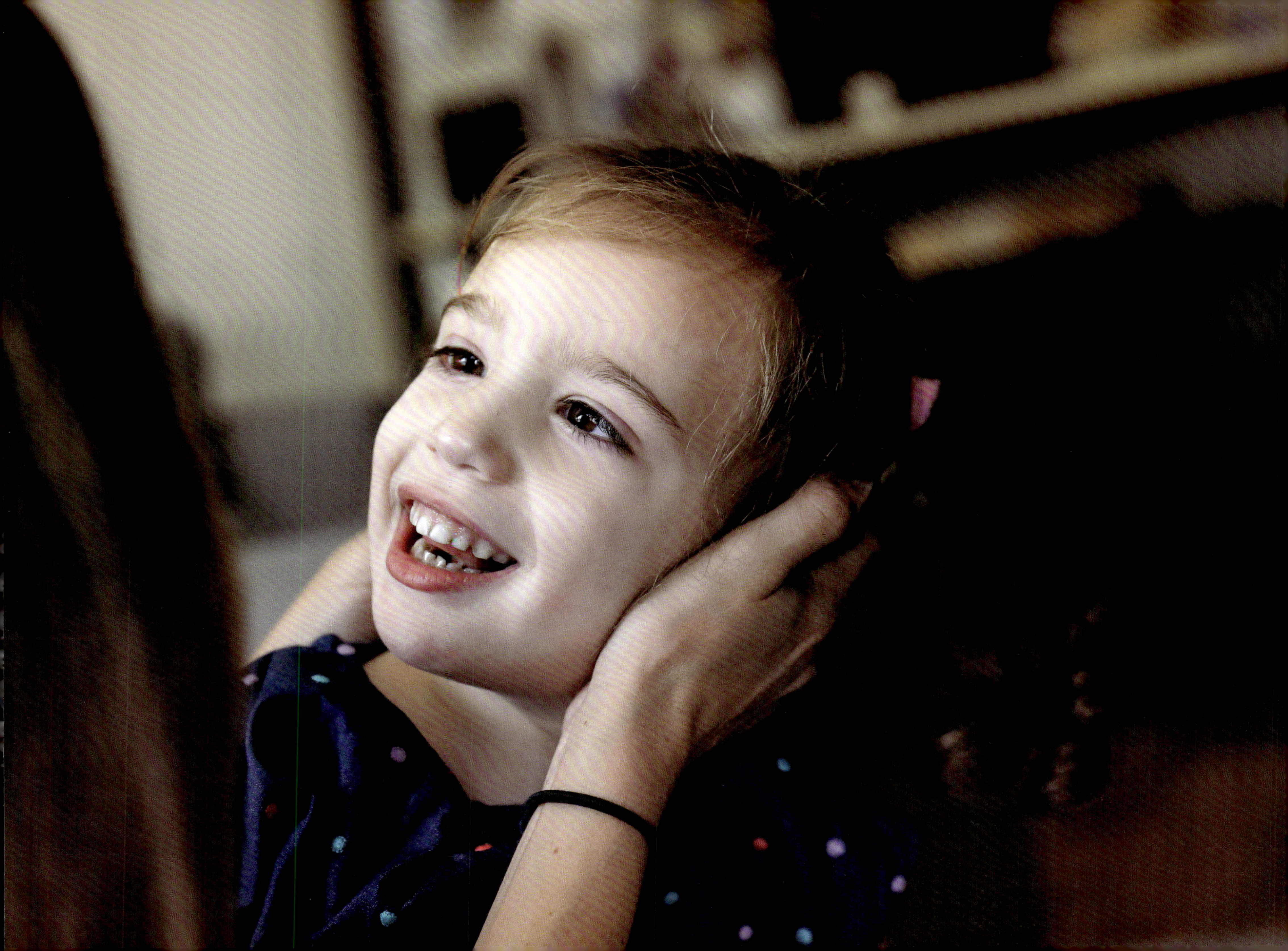

Last time I went for blood work, I was walking into the place and I was thinking I'm going to be scared. Then I was like "I can't be out-toughed by my four-year- old sister." I walked in, and I was like just do it. – Tanner, Josie's brother

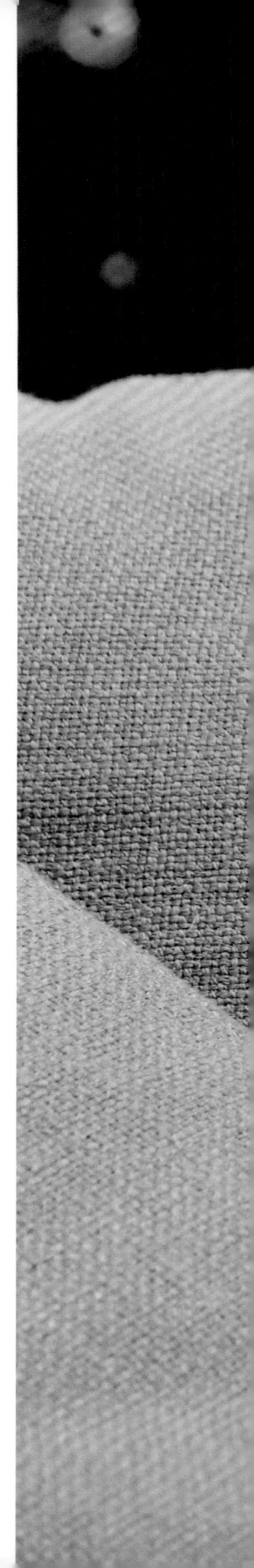

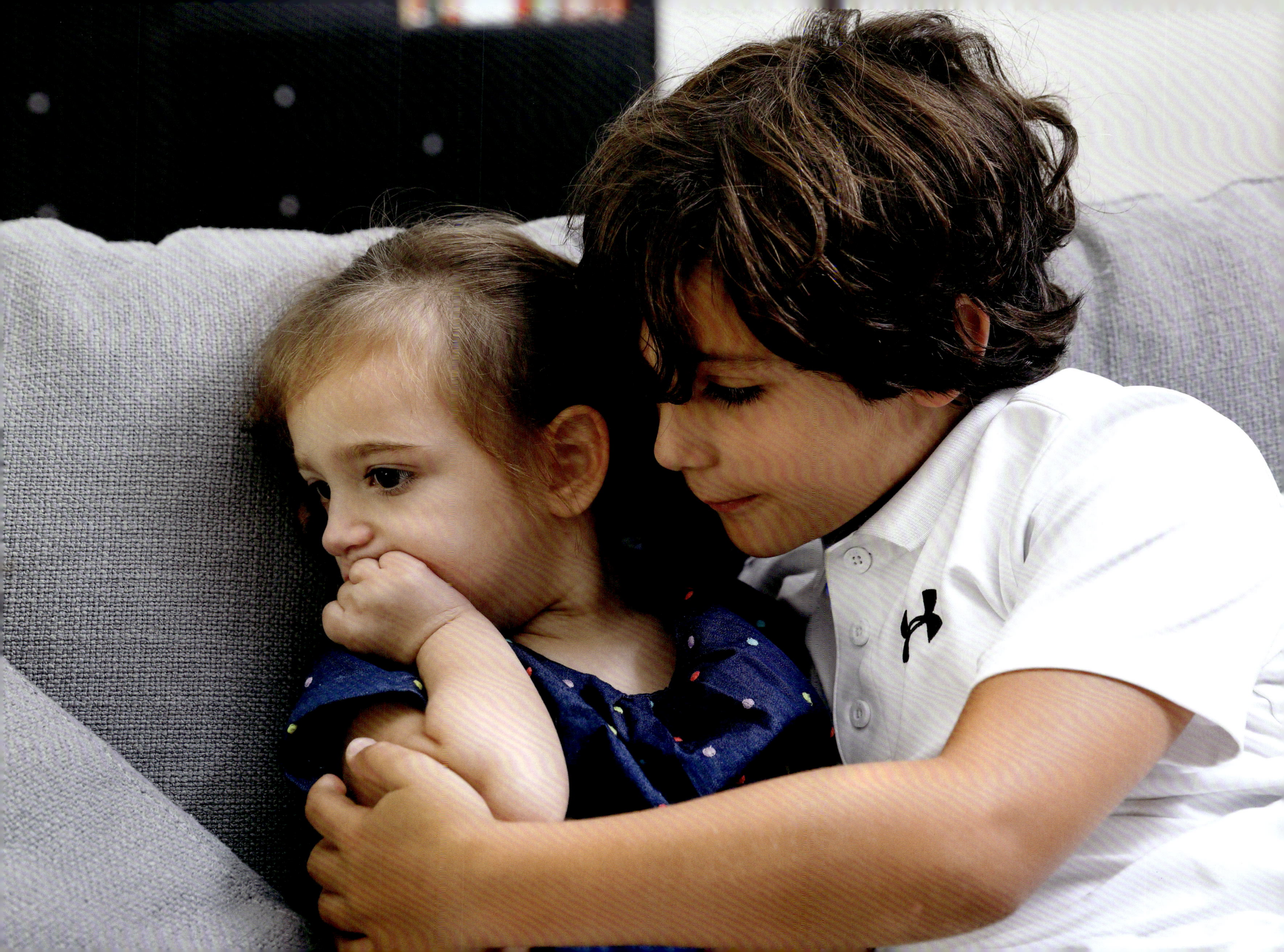

In 5th grade I got kind of depressed over my illness and I thought I was alone in everything. We went to therapy and she helped me write a blog that she wanted me to do, and then she kind of gave us little ideas to start Fighting H.A.R.D. for other kids. That was kind of my outlet from the depression—to help other kids to not feel that way, because I knew that was not a good feeling.
– Alexandra

Alexandra & Jonna

Alexandra, 13, and Jonna, 12, both suffer from chronic illnesses. Alexandra battles chronic inflammation, which has caused Crohn's disease, juvenile rheumatoid arthritis, and joint inflammation throughout her body. Meanwhile, at the age of 11, Jonna's stomach muscles essentially stopped working—a condition known as gastroparesis. Inspired by their own struggles with sickness, the sisters founded Fighting H.A.R.D., a foundation that seeks to help children with chronic illnesses and rare diseases. Jonna loves to play soccer when she is feeling well. She also enjoys watching cooking shows. Alexandra loves music, art, and writing in her spare time.

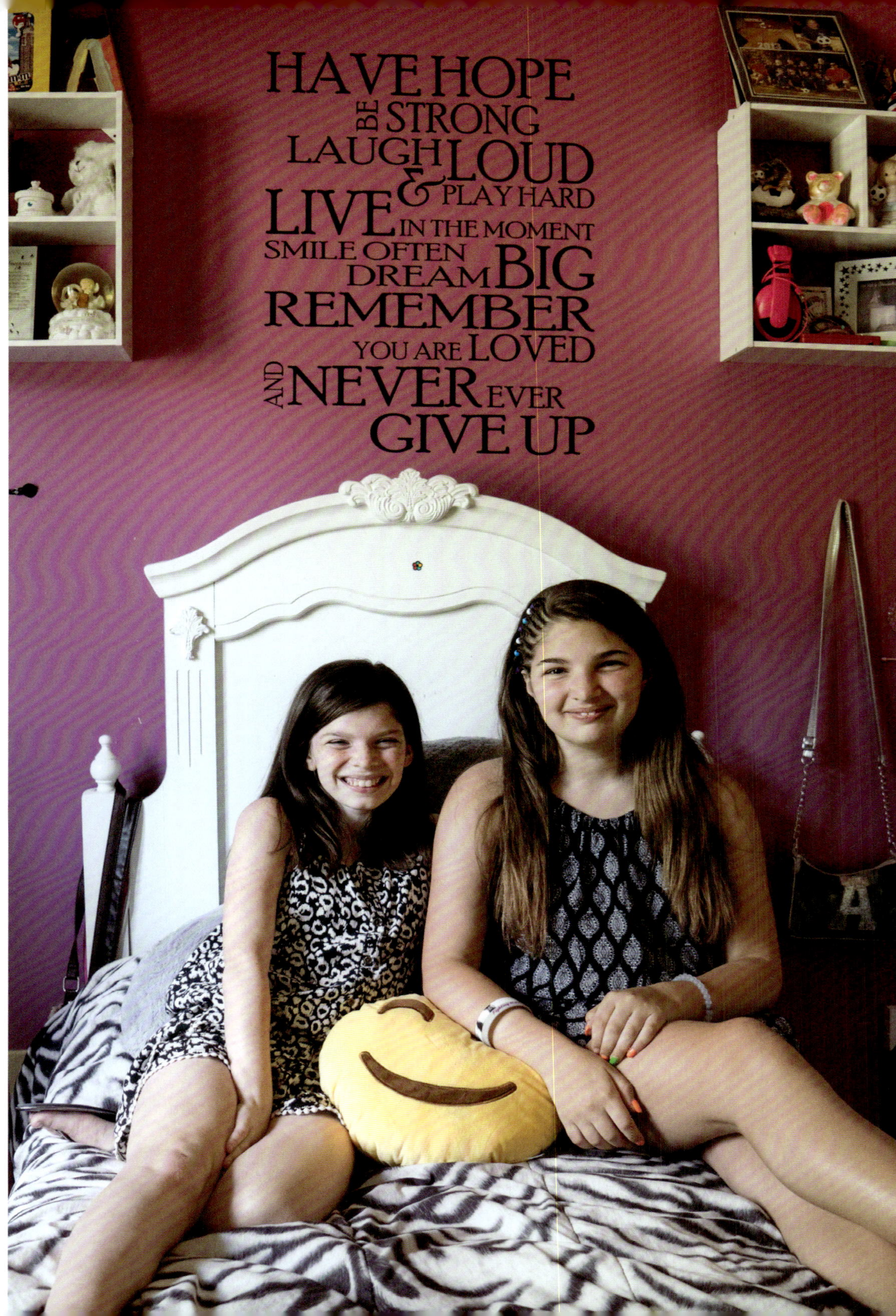
HAVE HOPE
BE STRONG
LAUGH LOUD
& PLAY HARD
LIVE IN THE MOMENT
SMILE OFTEN
DREAM BIG
REMEMBER
YOU ARE LOVED
AND NEVER EVER
GIVE UP

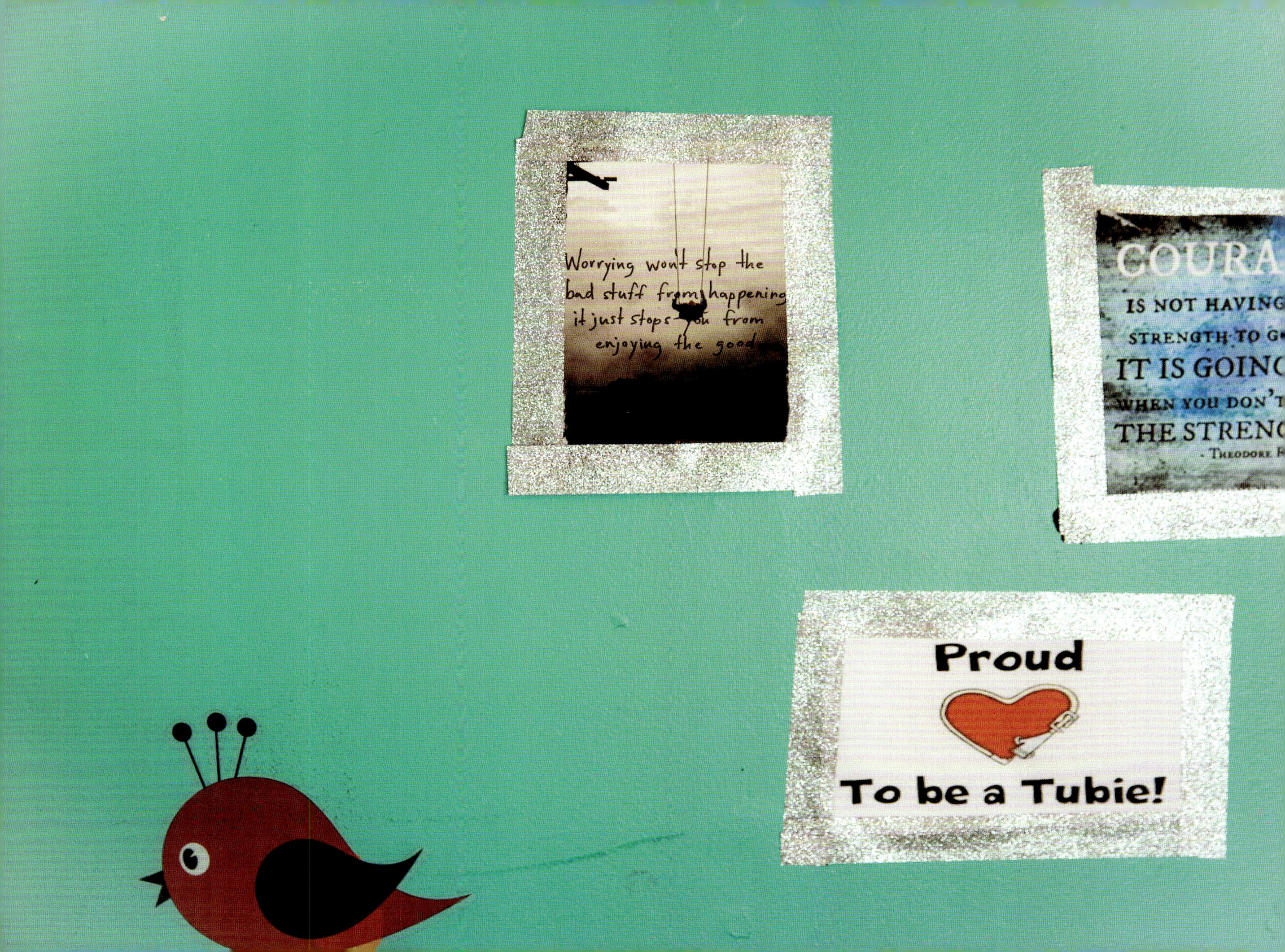
Worrying won't stop the bad stuff from happening it just stops you from enjoying the good
IS NOT HAVING
STRENGTH TO G
IT IS GOING
WHEN YOU DON'T
THE STRENG
Proud
To be a Tubie!

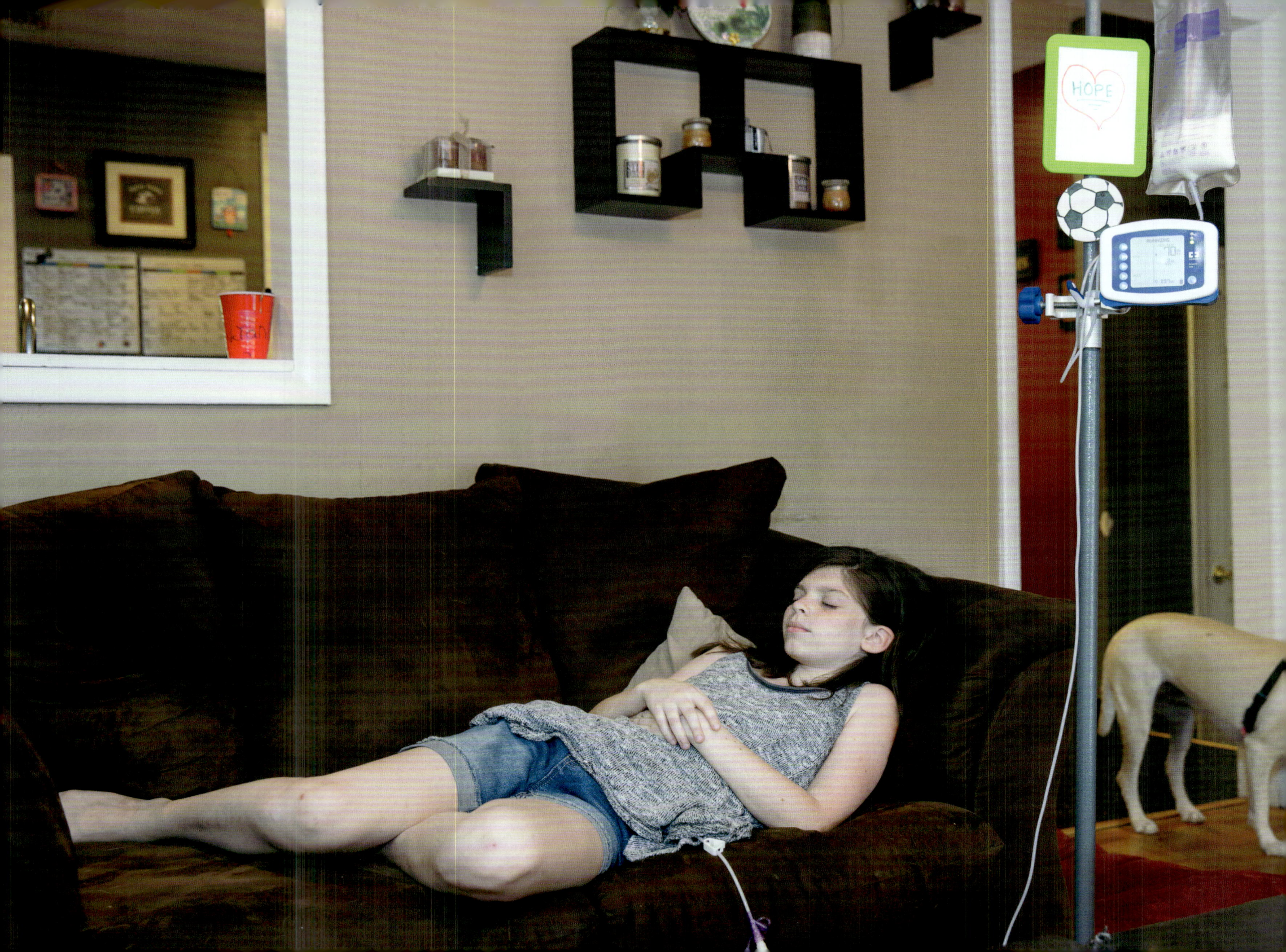
HOPE

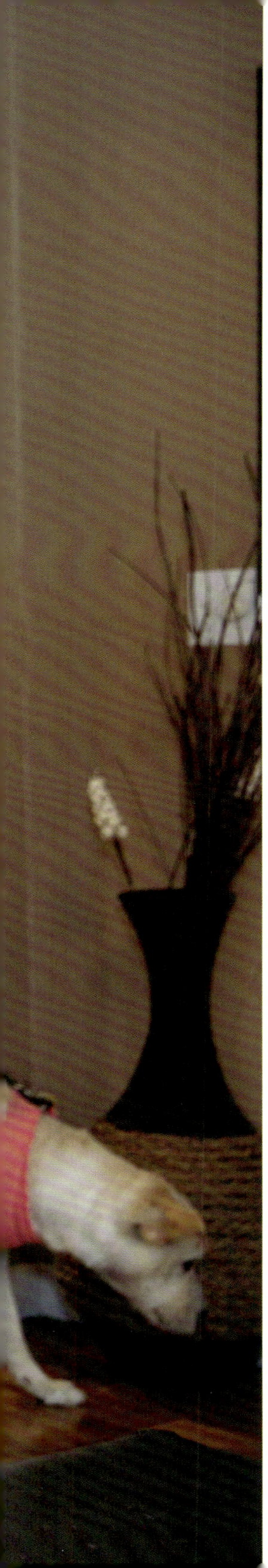

JONNA REQUIRES A FEEDING TUBE FOR ALL HER NOURISHMENT.

You try not take the little things for granted. Some smaller things, like when I drive home from work, her car's in the driveway, that's something that makes me pretty happy. I come home, I hear the Wii going. A lot of times, that doesn't happen. They are in the hospital for months at a time sometimes. Not to have everyone here, is kind of a big deal, so when I do come home and everyone is here, or things are as normal as they can be, it's just everyday life, I'm not taking that for granted, it's fully appreciated.
– Jon, Alexandra and Jonna's father

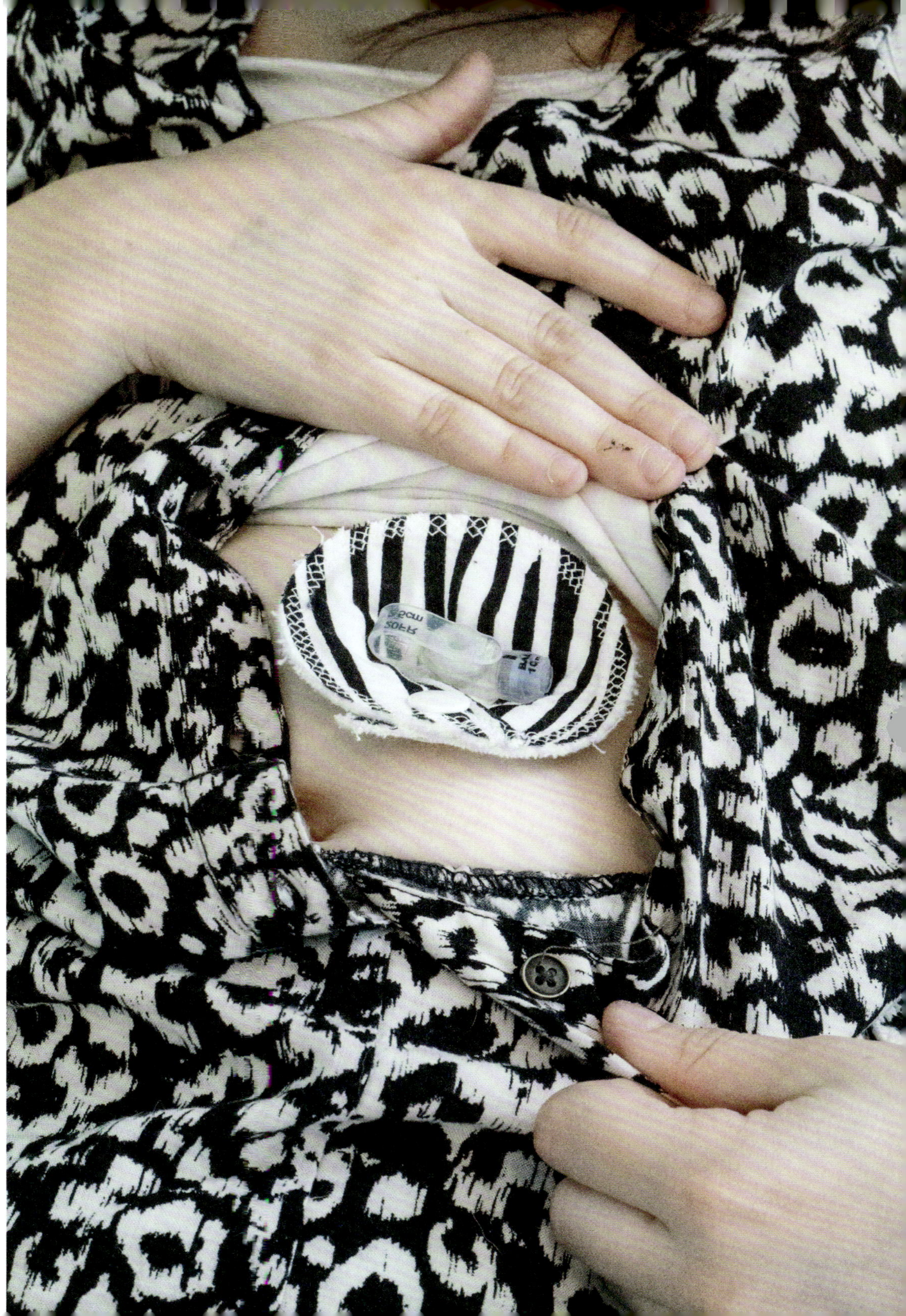

We send out little Play-Doh packages to kids, all of our Fighting H.A.R.D. kids and so they make things and they can send pictures to us so they can show us what they made. And when they're in the hospital or when they're not feeling good, it really helps them to be happier and have something fun to do. – Jonna

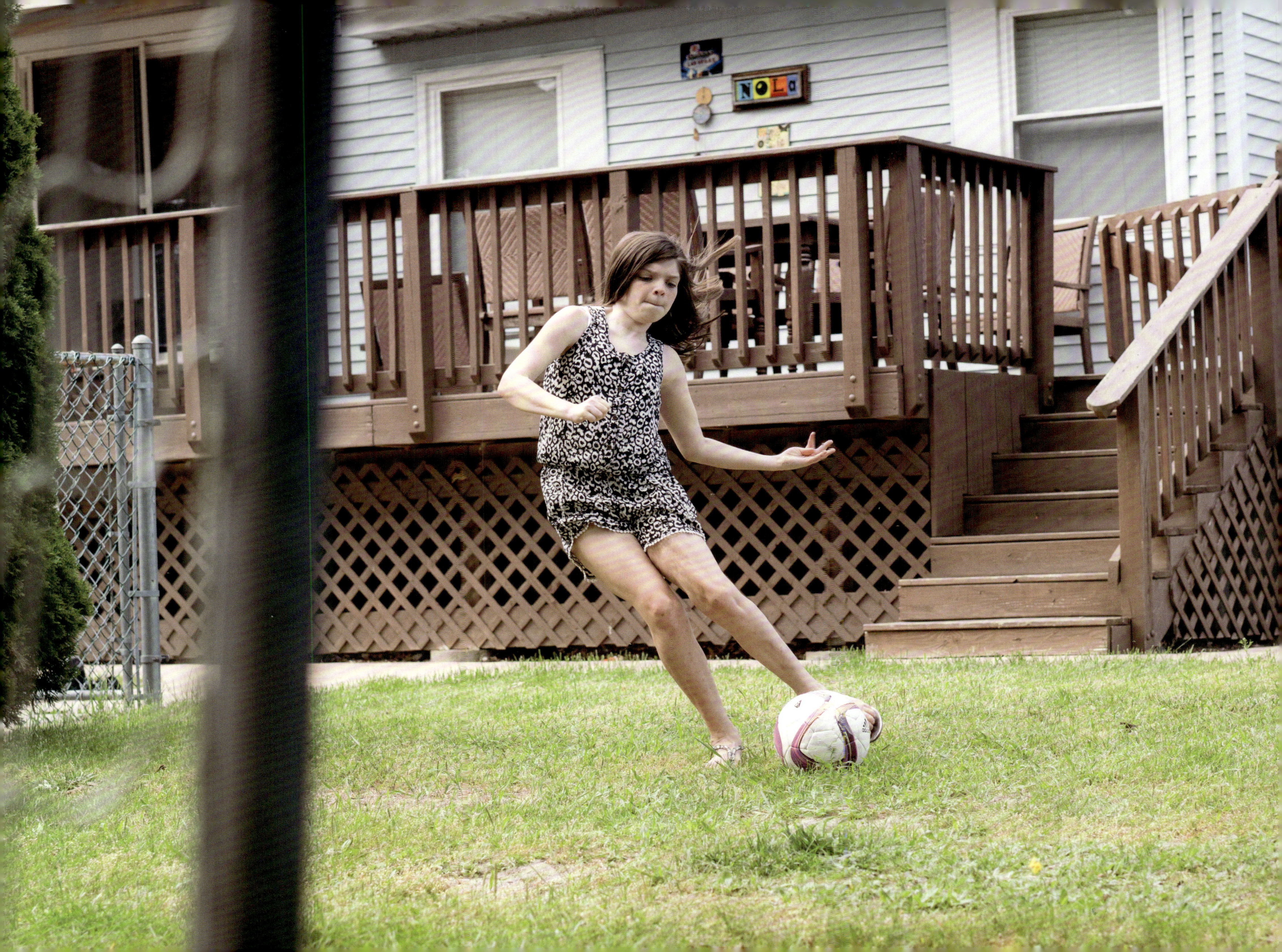
NOLa

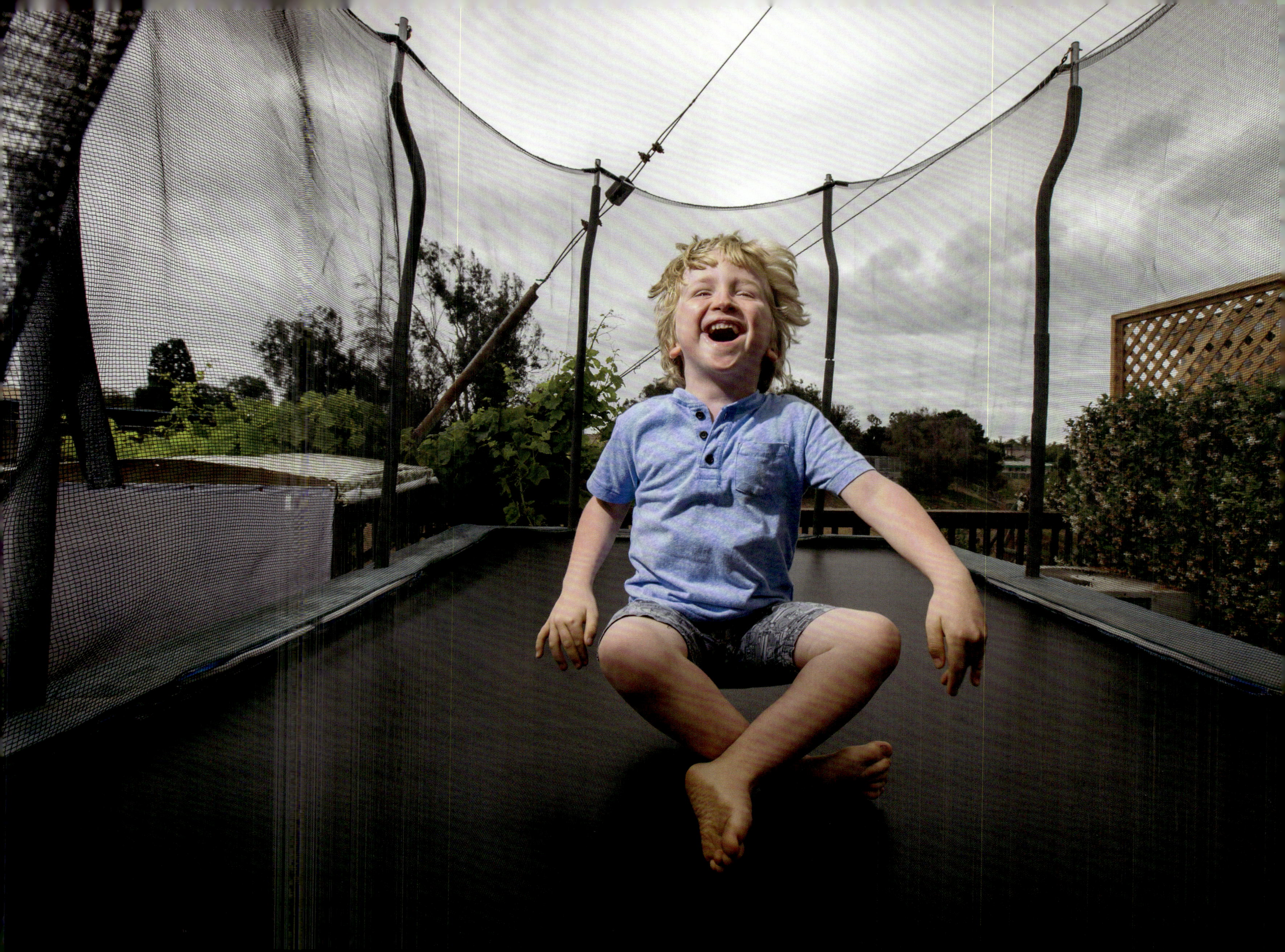

Ian

According to Ian's dad it was, "Pretty much game on as soon as he was born." Ian, 5, required full-time oxygen for the first three years of his life and was later diagnosed with Megalencephaly-capillary malformation syndrome [MCAP], and Polymicrogyria [PMG]. Symptoms vary from patient to patient but for Ian it includes a large head, body asymmetry, developmental delays, soft skin which gets red or blue from change in temperature, seizures, and low muscle tone. Ian loves books, sensory items like beans and rocks, Thomas the train, and singing with his mom.

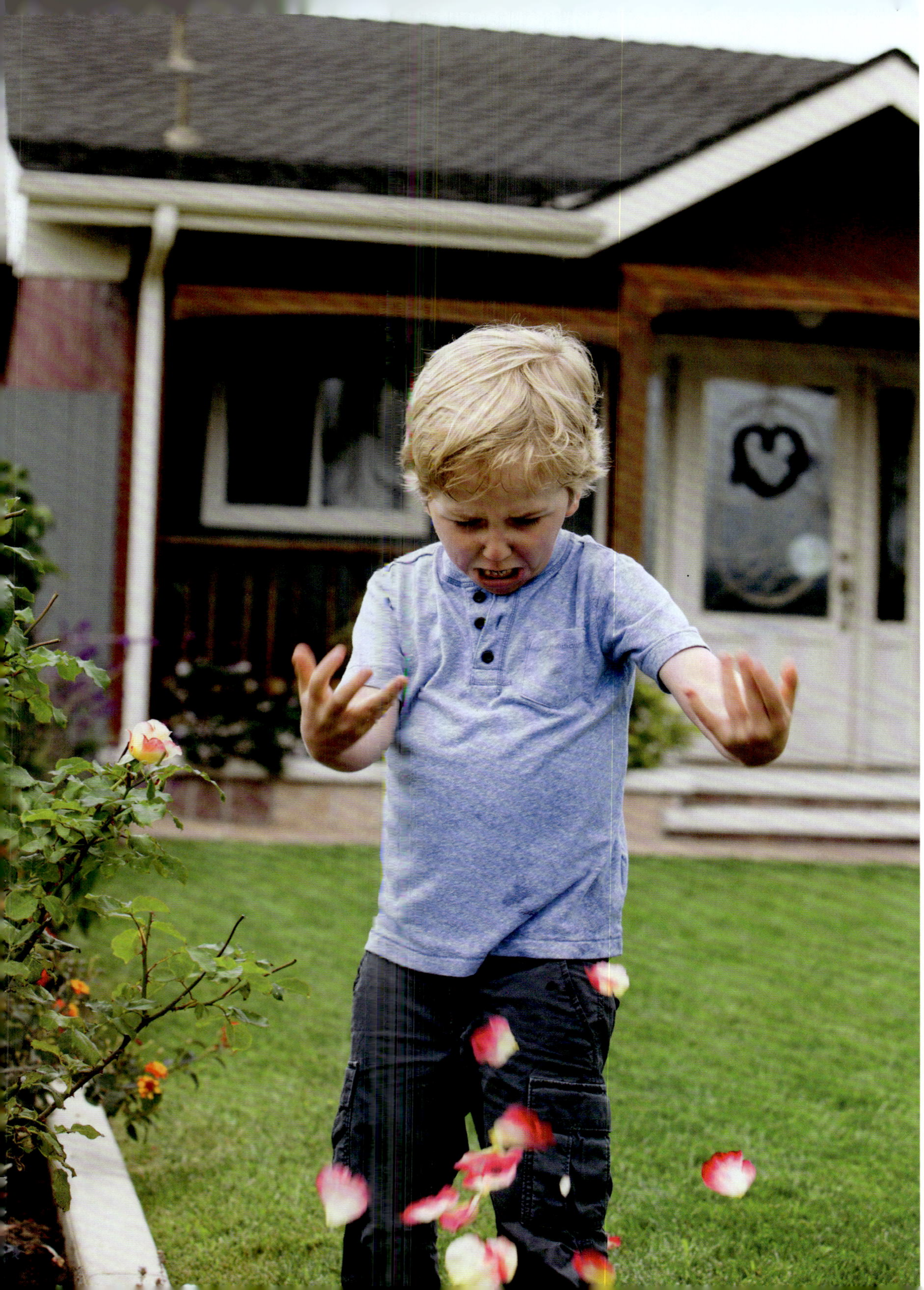

Most of these kids will eat and eat and eat and they don't realize that they're full. They'll just keep eating. They cannot get satiated. – Shari, Ian's mother

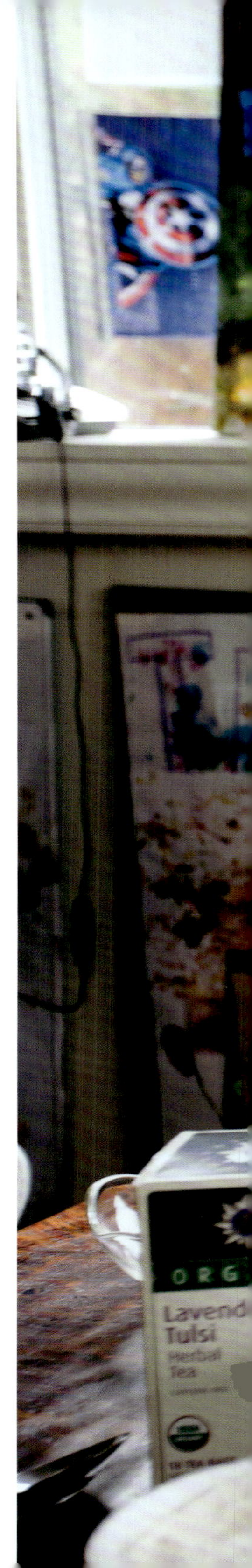

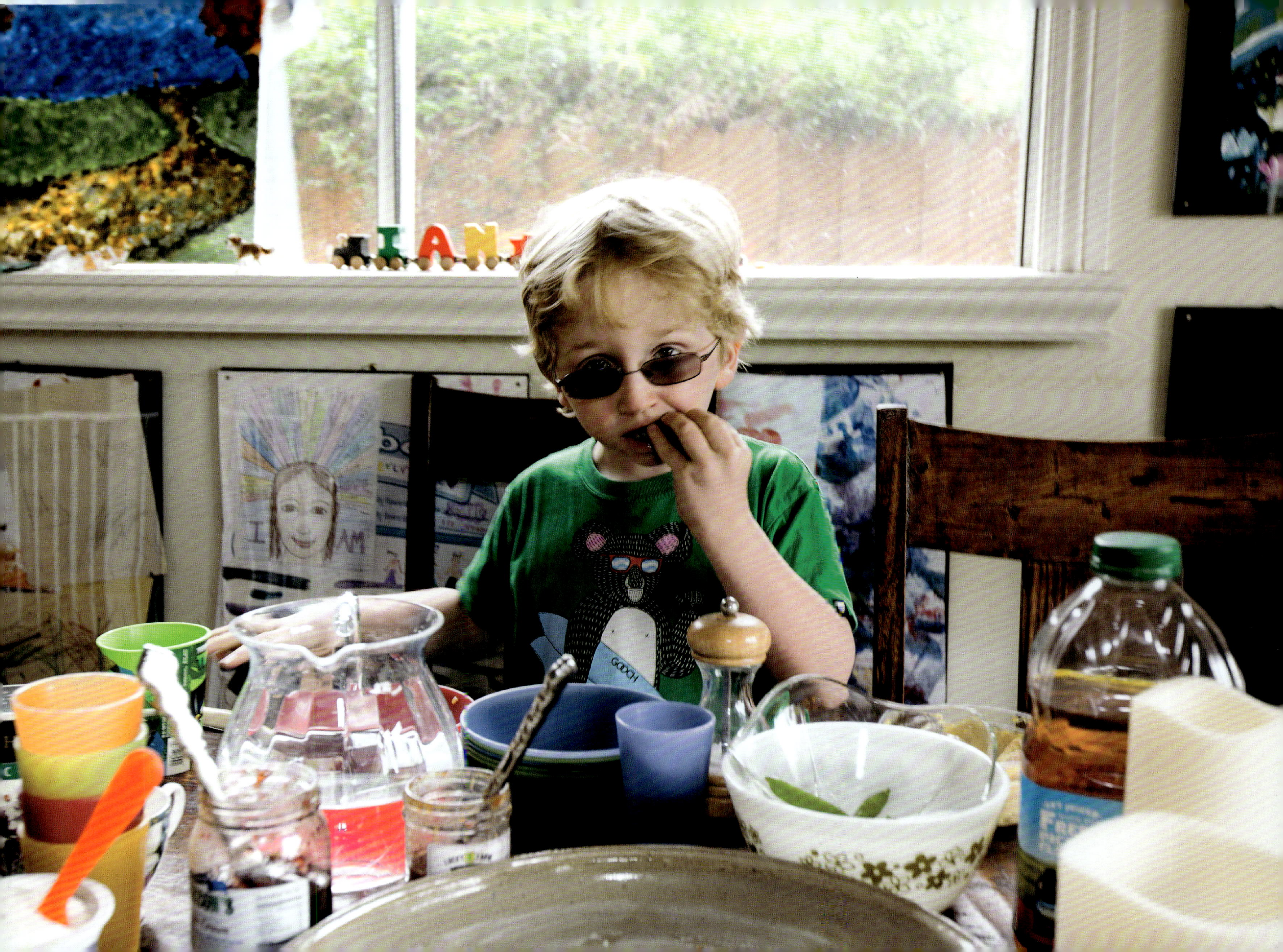
I AM

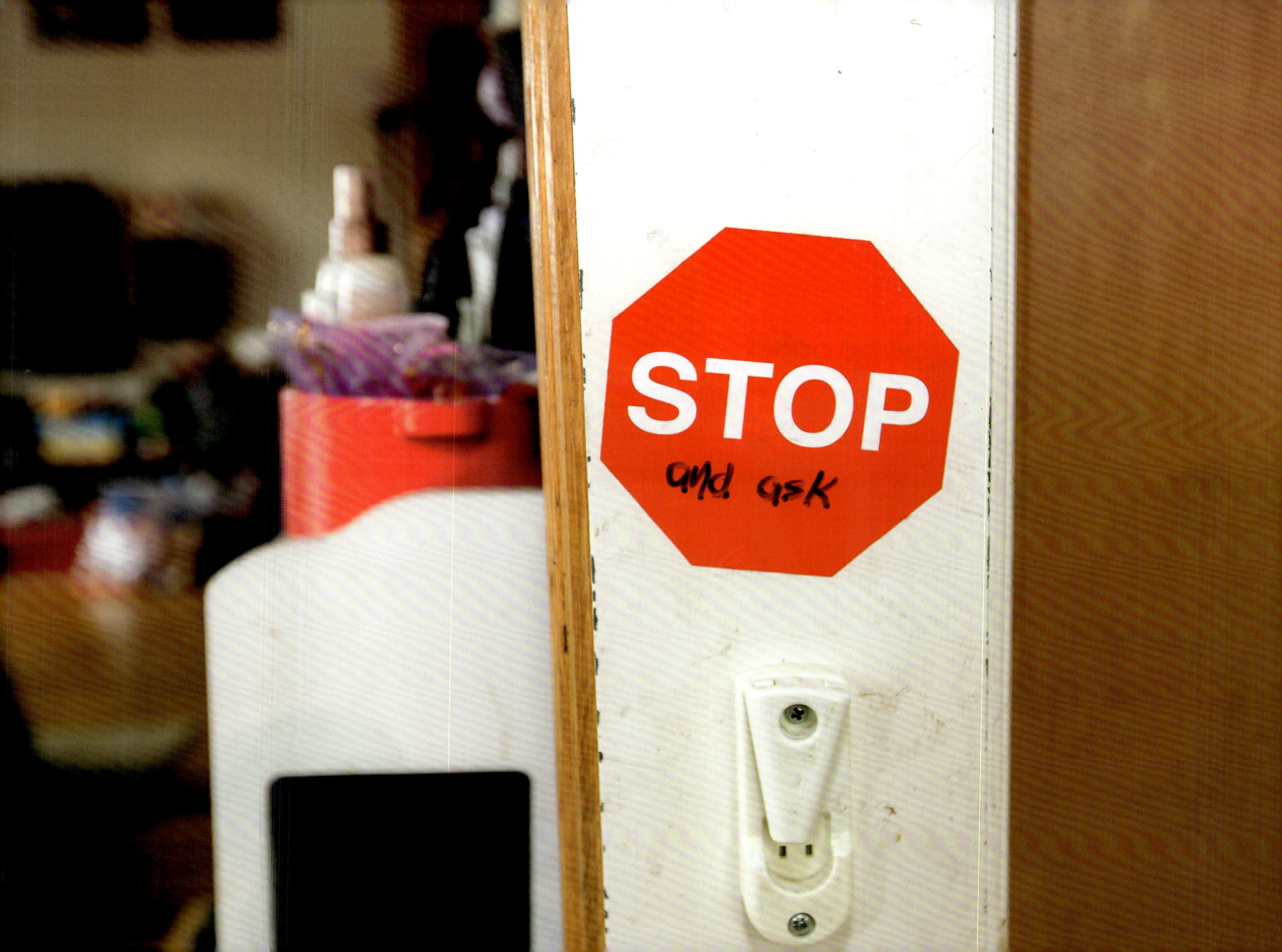
STOP
and ask

REMINDER SIGNS ARE NEEDED THROUGHOUT THE HOUSE TO PROTECT IAN. A STOP SIGN ON THE FRIDGE DISCOURAGES HIM FROM OVEREATING.

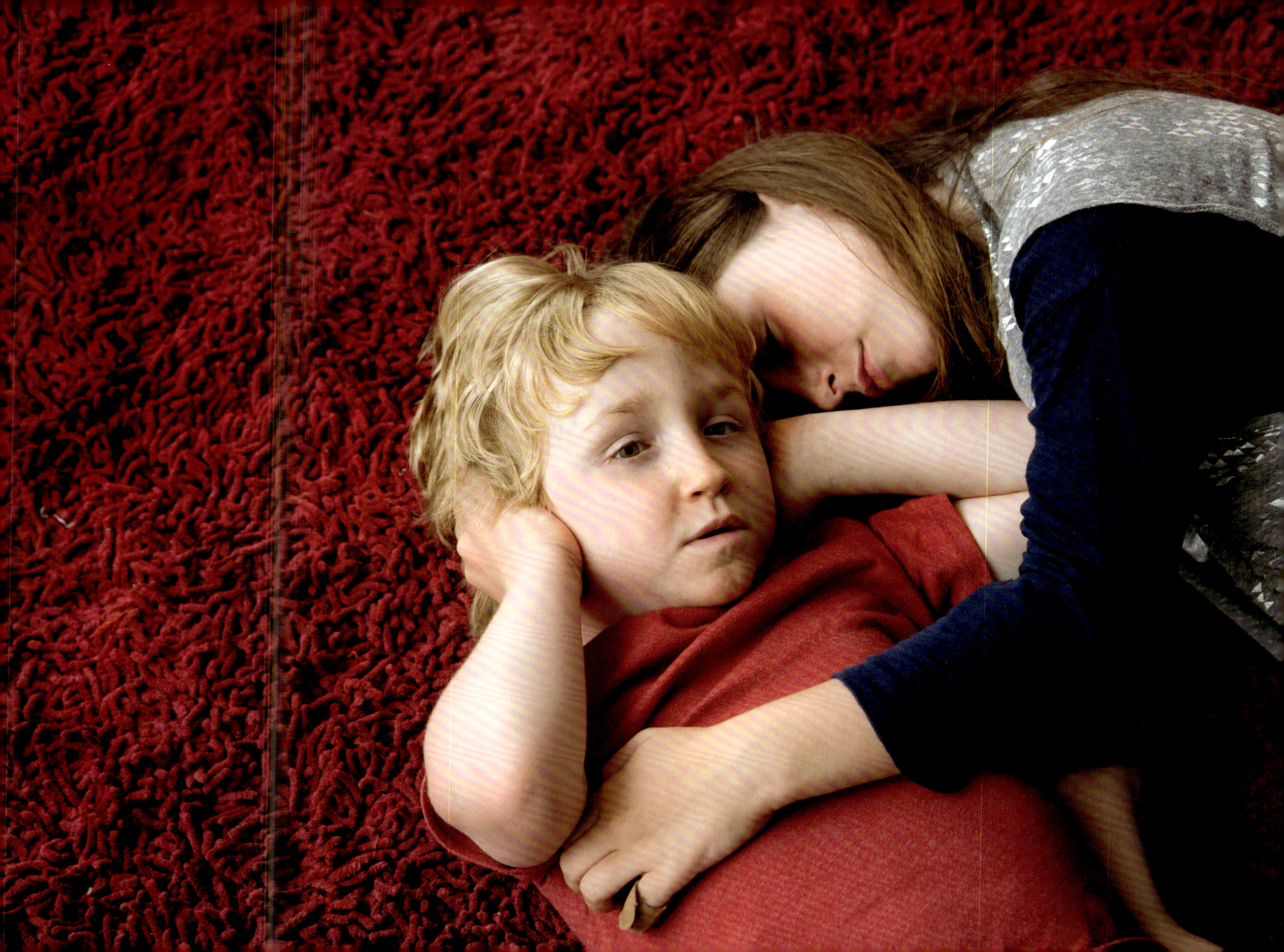

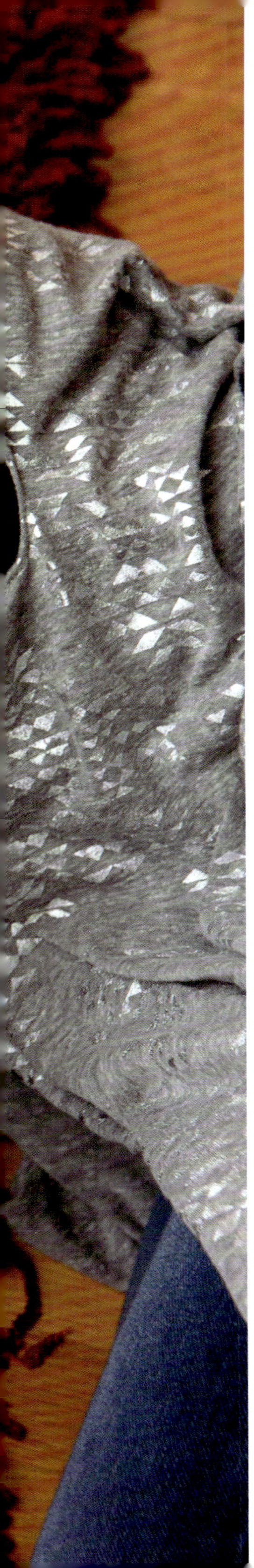

People need to know what's going on with these kids. They need to know, "Okay, there's going to be kids in this world that can't do what I can do. What can I do to help them?" – Lila, Ian's sister

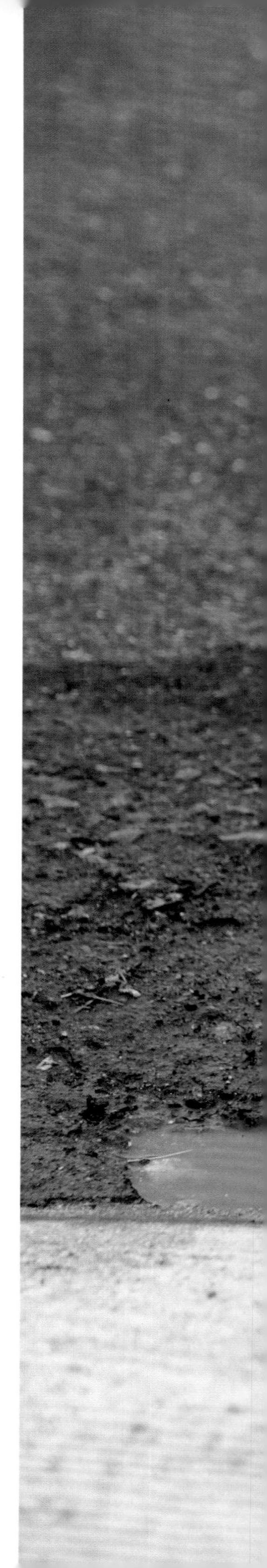

It's a challenge...allowing him to be a child and play and be his fun self in the very limited amount of time during the day that he has where he's not in therapy or in school. – Shari, Ian's mother

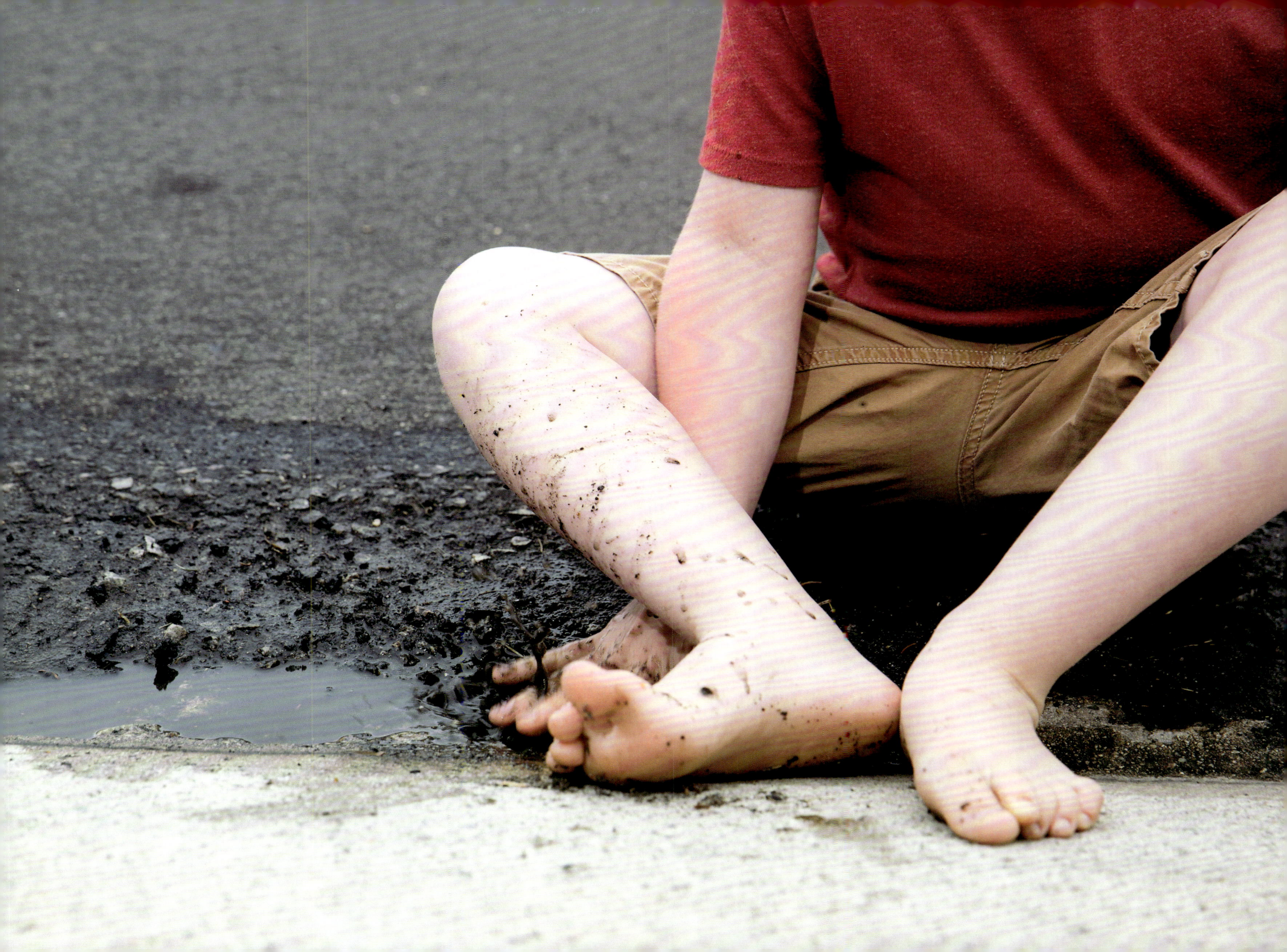

It can happen to anybody. It does change your world, it does change your lifestyle, but with support systems and whatnot, you get through it and you make the best of it. – Michelle, Quinn's mother

Quinn

Quinn, 5, has polymicrogyria, which, in her case, consists of wrinkles on the left side of her brain. This condition causes seizures, developmental delays, and problems with speech and swallowing. Recently, Quinn began speaking a little. She loves cars, playing ball, trampolines, music, and dancing.

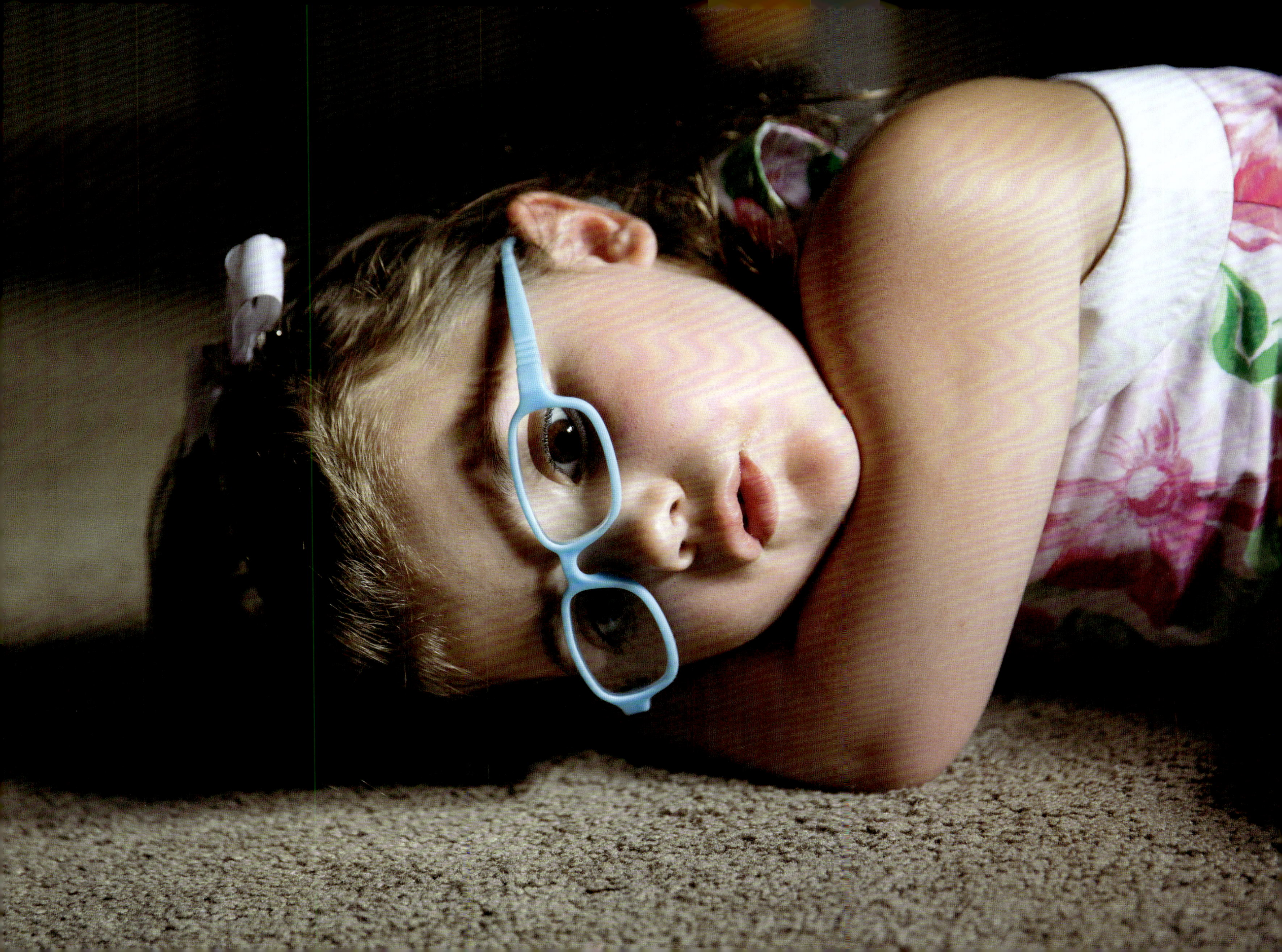

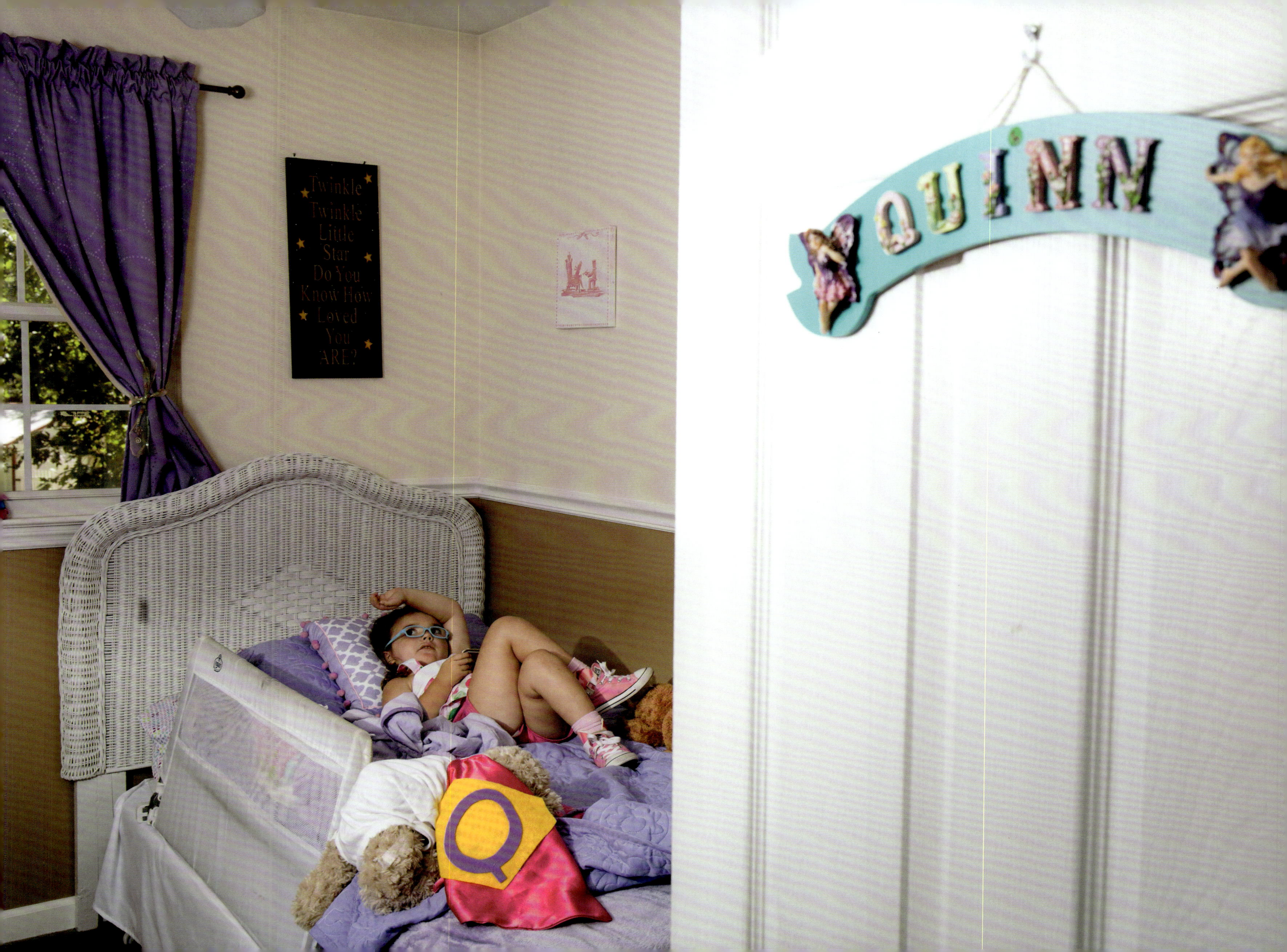
Twinkle
Twinkle
Little
Star
Do You
Know How
Loved
You
ARE?
QUINN
Q

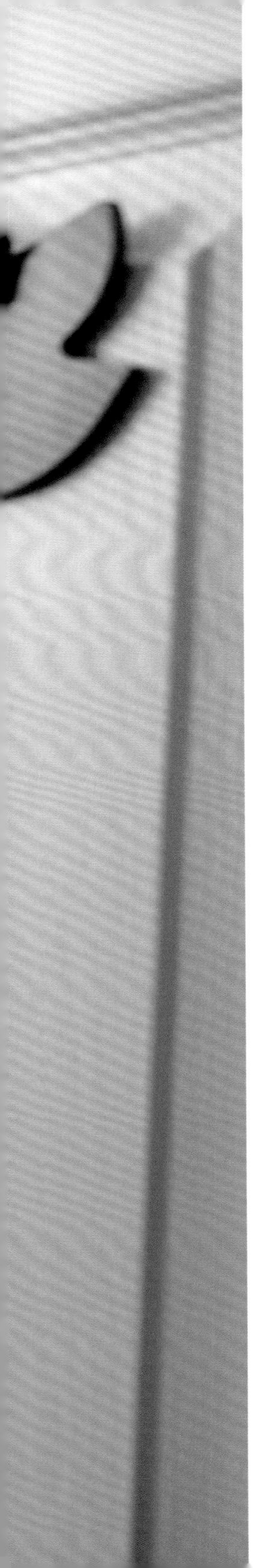

They basically said, "We don't know much about this. We don't know if she will ever walk. We don't know if she will ever talk. We don't know if she will ever eat on her own."
– Michelle, Quinn's mother

She is writing her own book. So far she is writing a really good story.
– Michelle, Quinn's mother

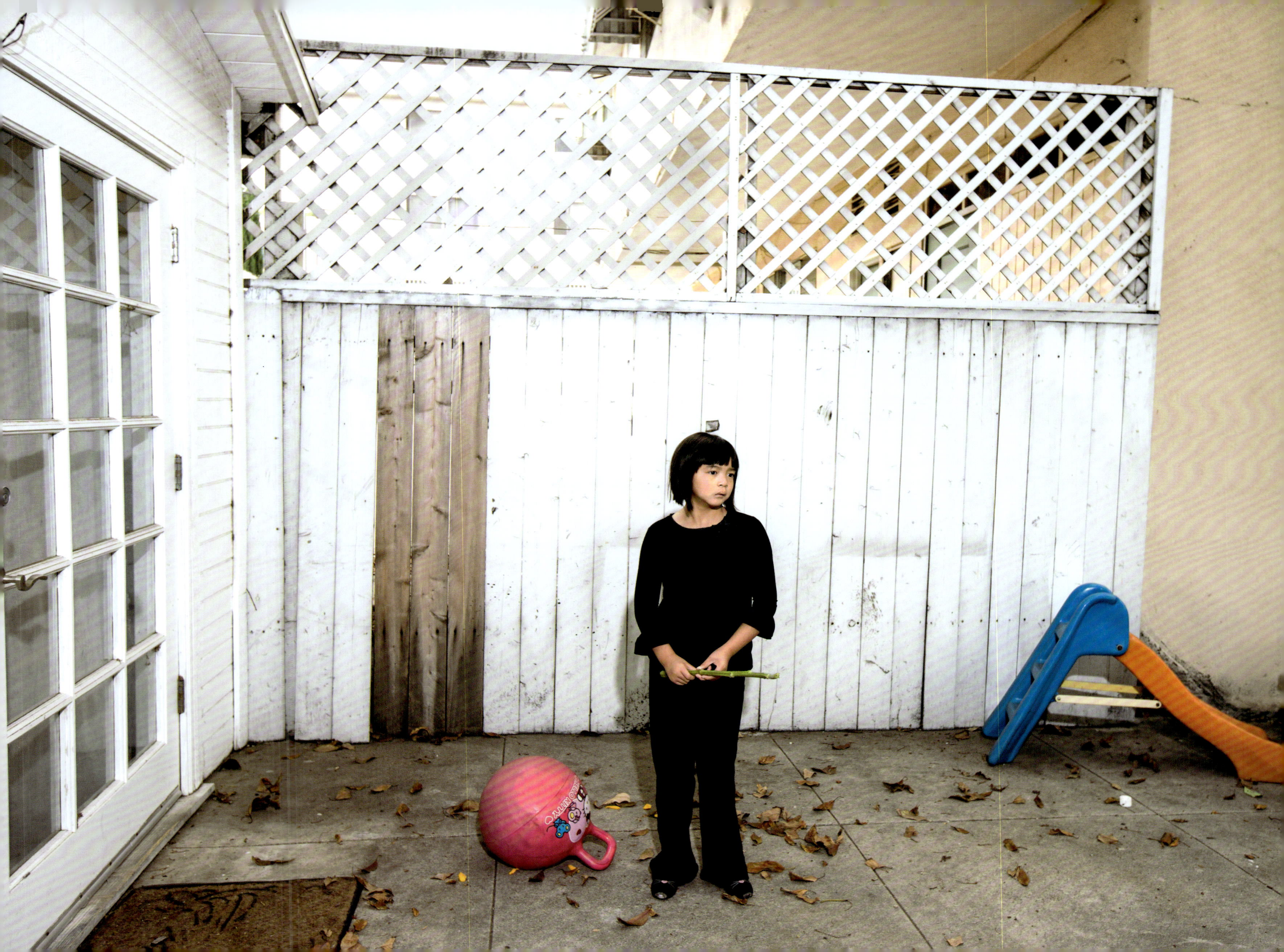

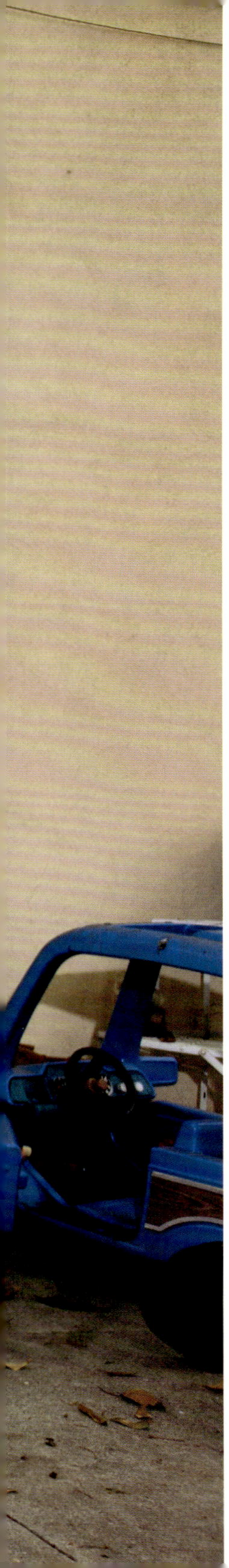

It's so rare, the technology had just been developed to be able to discover something like that, so there's no name. There's not a history, and the medical genetic doctor said, "Well, it'll be very interesting following this little girl, because there's no road map."
– Lisa, Zoey's mother

Zoey

Zoey's parents adopted her from China with knowledge only of her cleft palate. Once significant developmental delays became apparent, doctors determined that Zoey has chromosome deletion syndrome of the 2Q32 chromosome—a condition so rare, it does not have a name. Zoey has learning disabilities and cognitive delays. She is 10 years old and is learning to write her name. Zoey loves her DVD player, phones, remotes, and things with buttons that she can press. She is often seen looking in the mirror or gazing at her reflection.

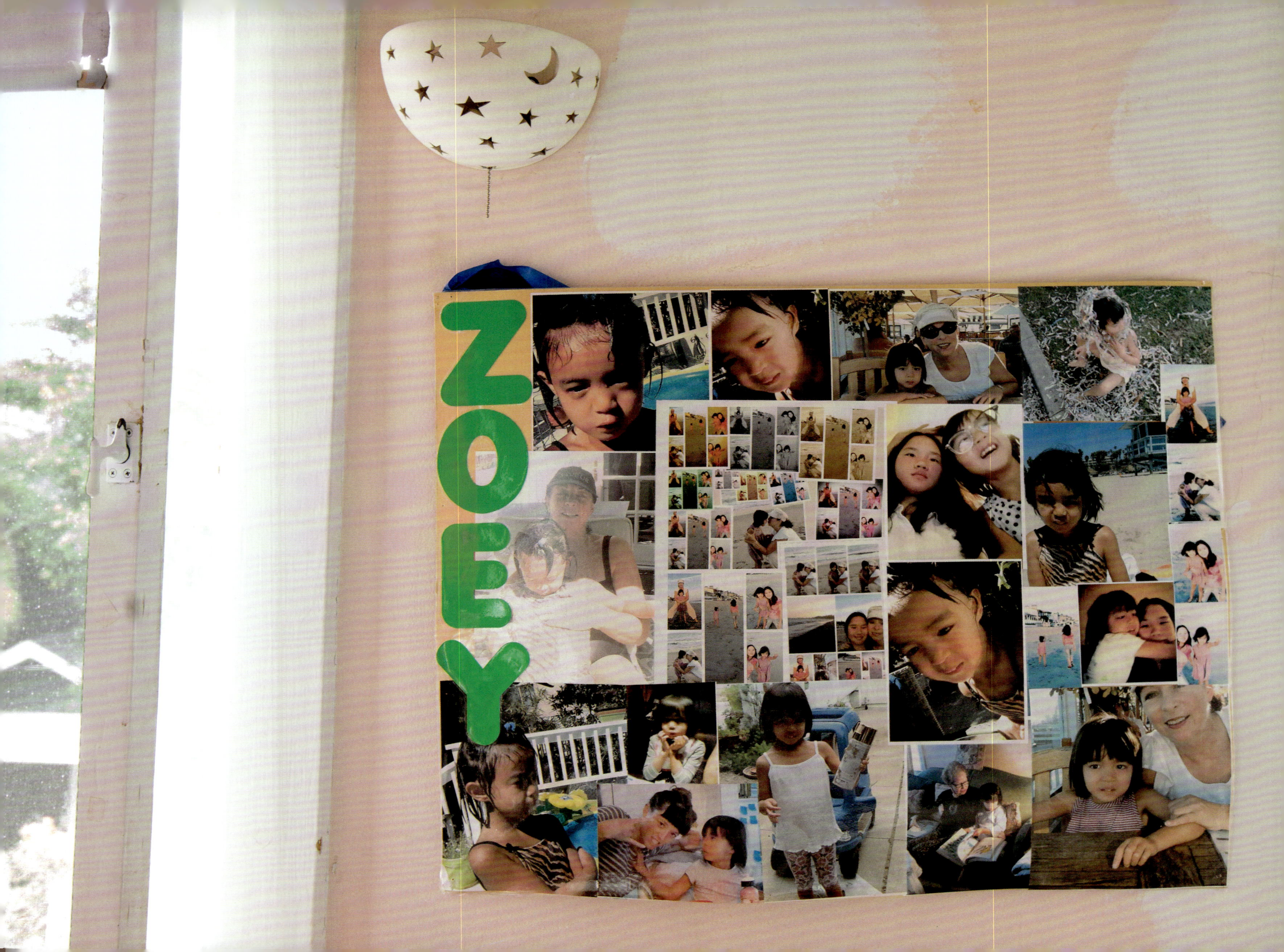
ZOEY

I have had her now for nine years, and I've certainly gotten to know her well. However, there's just so much that I don't know what's going on in there, since she doesn't have words. Sometimes, I get frustrated because she's frustrated. She is wanting something, or needing something, and I don't know what it is. A lot of times, I can figure it out, but when I can't it's really challenging.
– Lisa, Zoey's mother

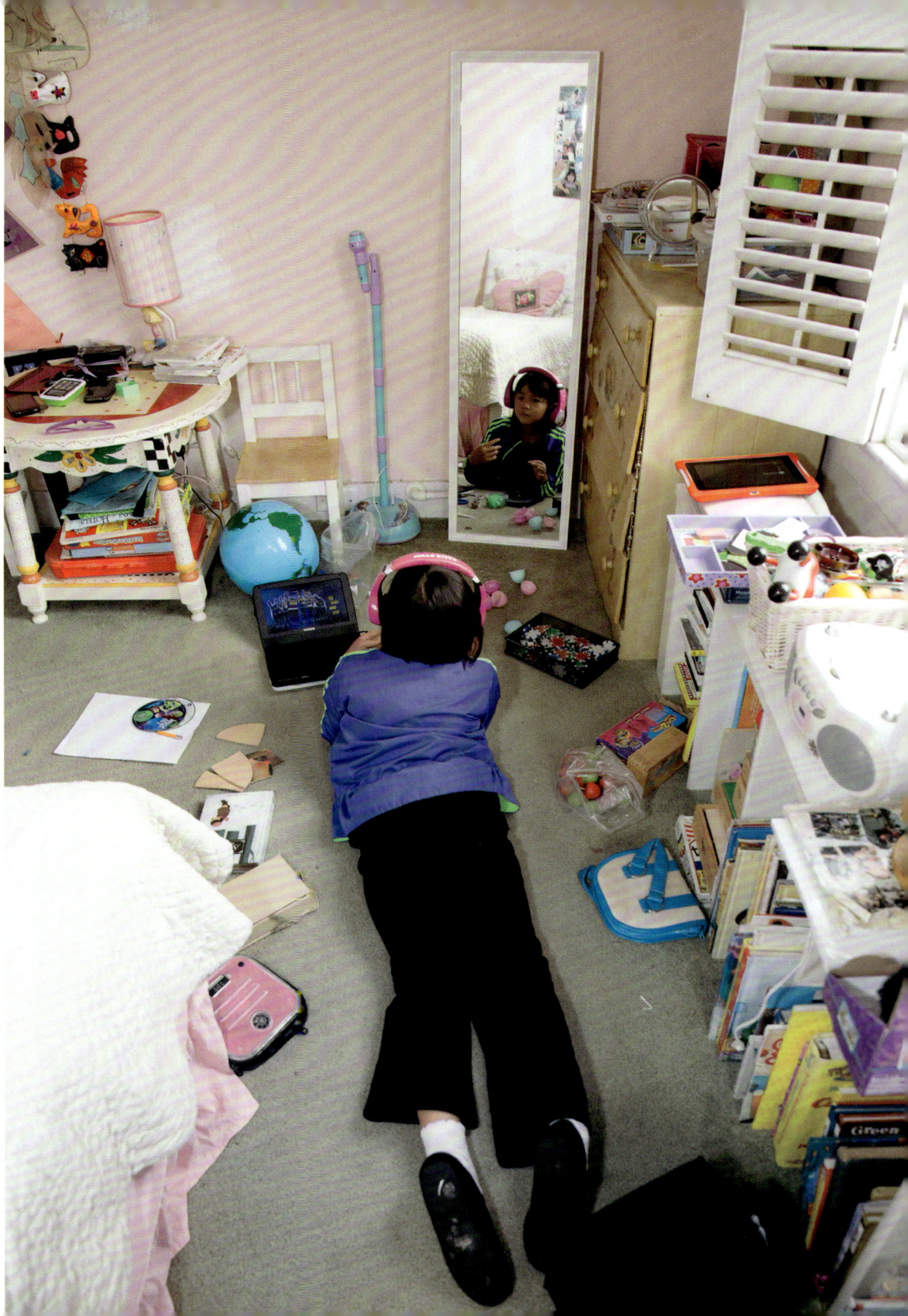

[My friends] don't make a big deal about it, because I don't say, "Here's my special needs sister." I just say, "This is Zoey. She'll follow us around." It's interesting, because you can't tell her to go. You can't be like, "Go in your room," or she'll follow, and then cry if she doesn't get what she wants. She gets pretty much everything she wants, when I'm around.
– Sophie, Zoey's sister

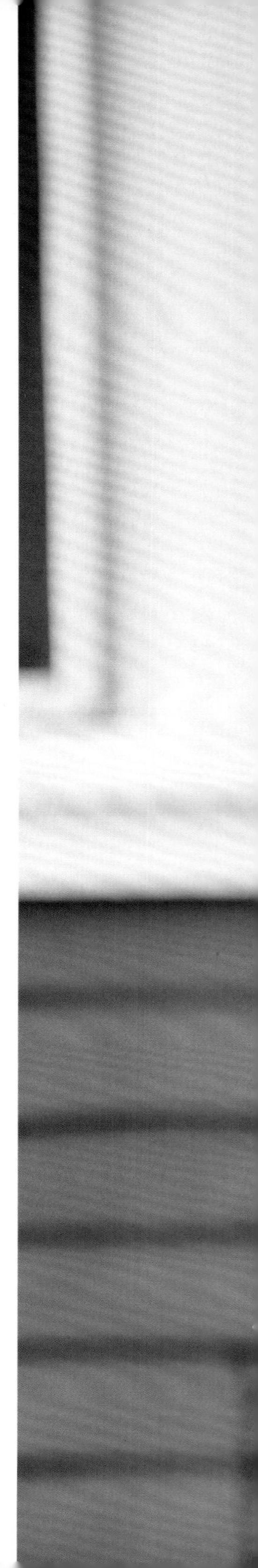

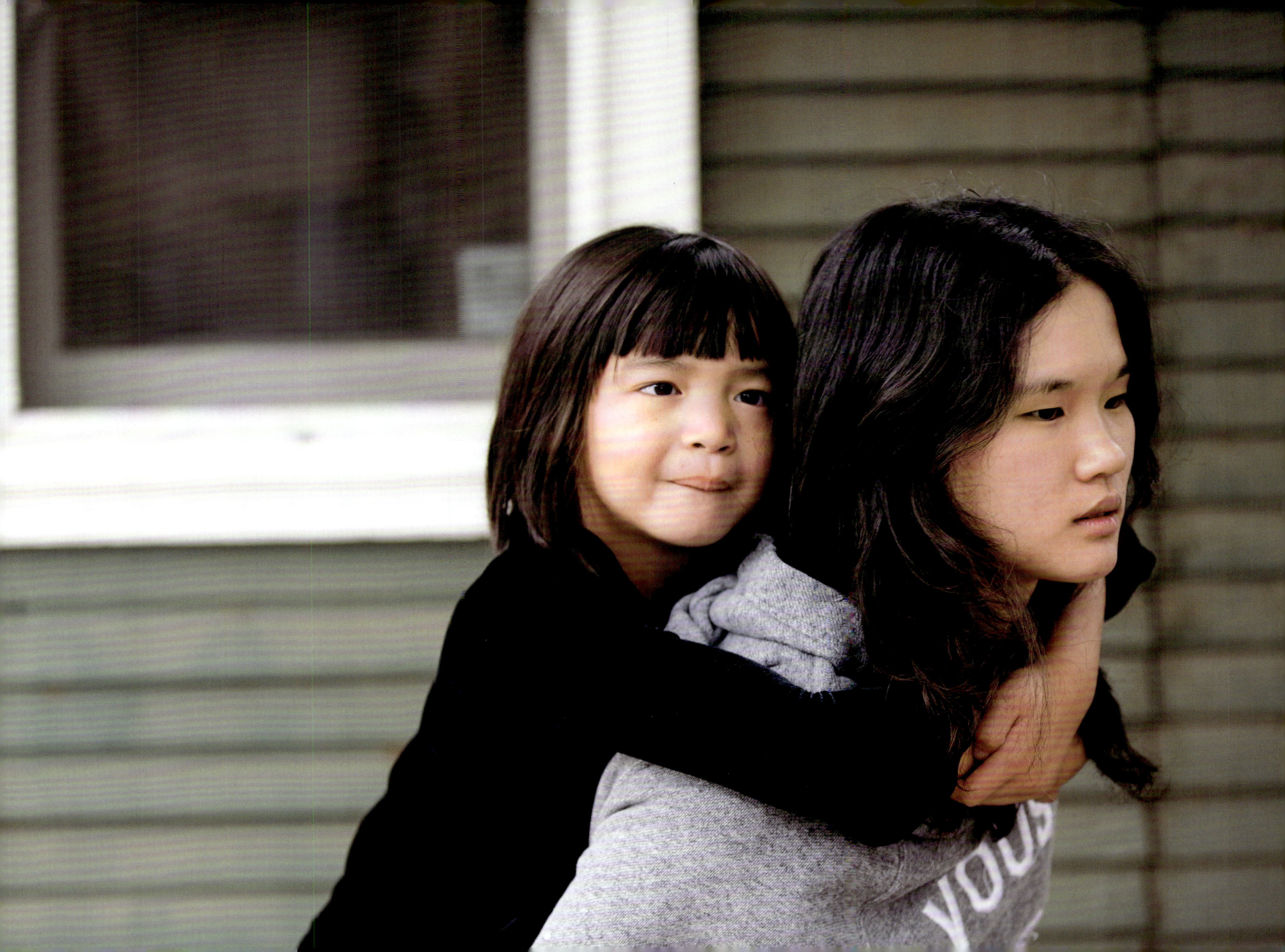

We have two children on the spectrum which makes it difficult to find a babysitter with the appropriate experience and comfort level in dealing with children on the spectrum. We are grateful that family and friends have offered to help but it's difficult for us just to let go. – Maria, Elena's mother

Elena

Elena, 6, has two genetic mutations. The first geneticist she saw at age two, told her parents there was "nothing significant to report" and not to worry. But at the age of 5 after additional genetic testing with a new geneticist, the tests showed that Elena has a mutation for autism and a rare mutation on the X chromosome known as BRWD3. Based on the limited number of persons with this mutation, symptoms may or may not include mild to moderate intellectual disability and macrocephaly. So far, Elena is the only known female with this mutation. Elena loves swinging in her backyard and likes looking at books.

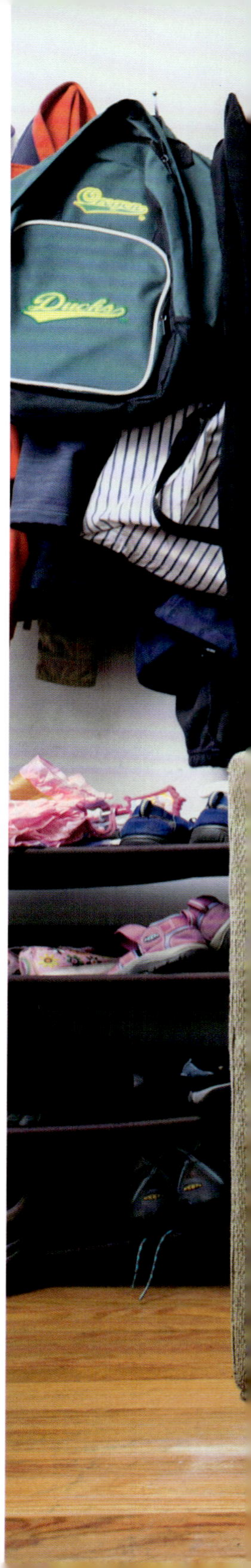

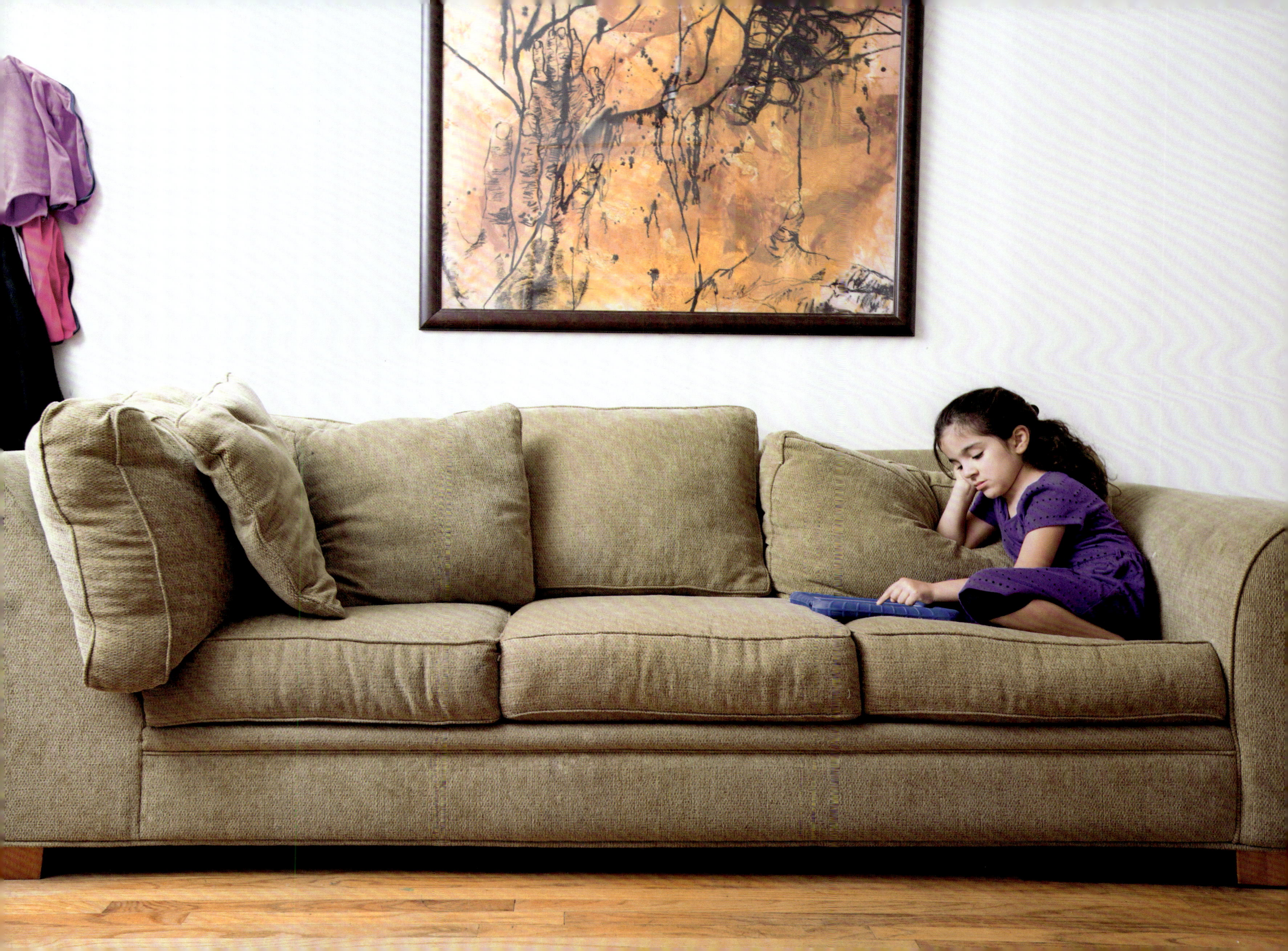

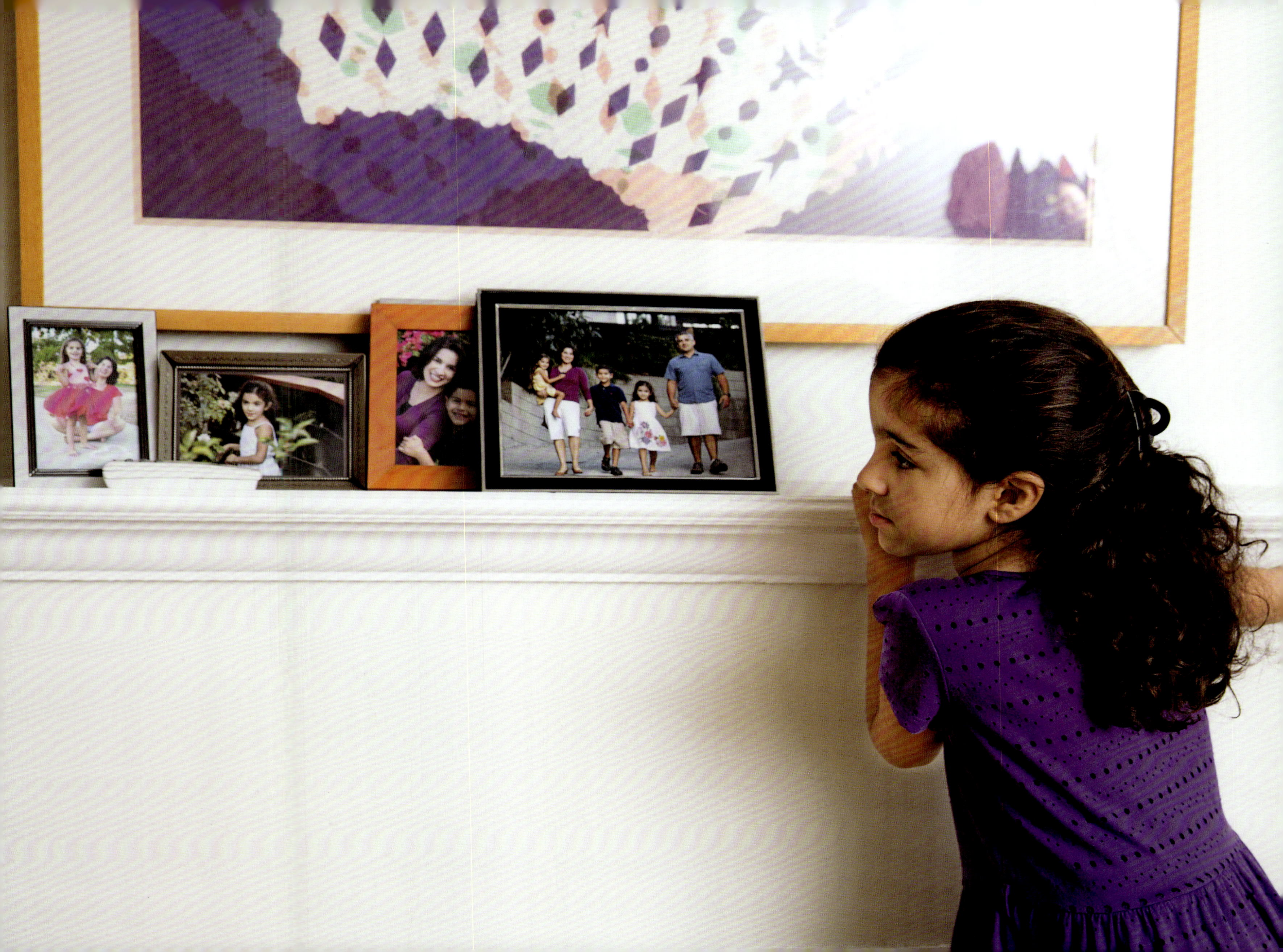

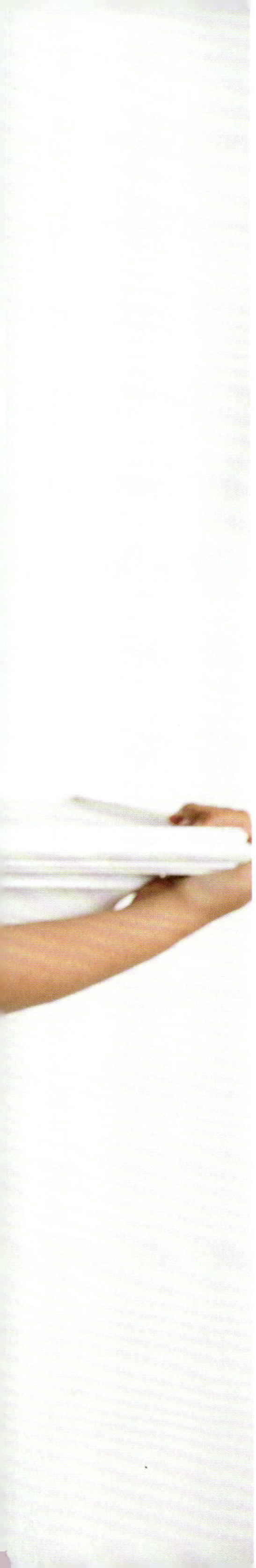

I think it's hardest for me knowing that my eldest son will spend the rest of his life taking care of his little sisters. I know that he feels alone. That's the toughest thing for me. – Argel, Elena's father

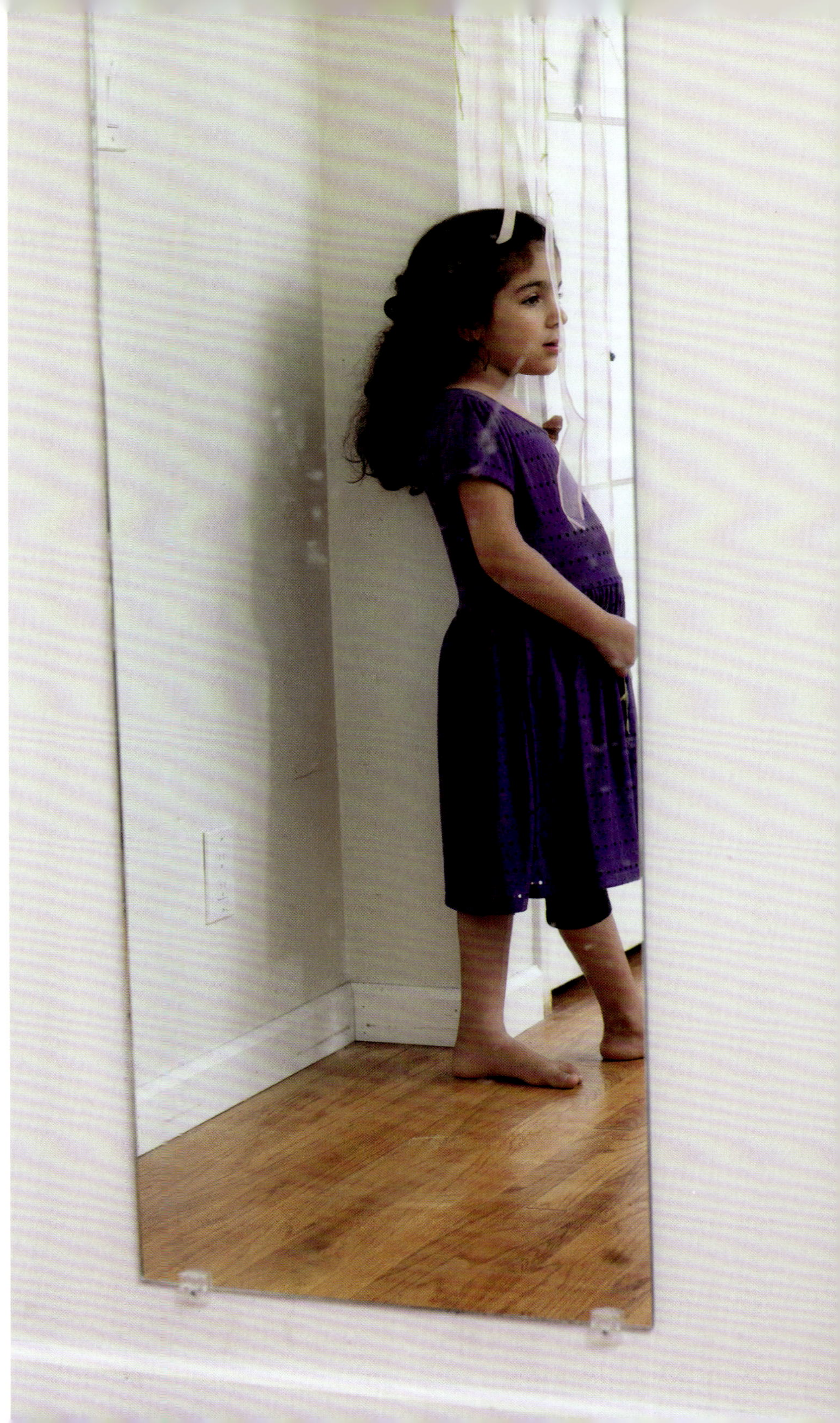

For six years, we thought she was an Autism Rett angel. Got very involved with the Rett community; we were doing walk-a-thons. [Her father] did golf outings, and made an entire family with the Rett syndrome moms and dads in New Jersey and all over the United States. – Elizabeth, Kelly's mother

Kelly

After three misdiagnoses, doctors concluded that Kelly suffers from a genetic mutation referred to most commonly as PACS1 syndrome, or as Schuurs-Hoeijmakers syndrome. At the time of her diagnosis, there were only three or four known cases in the United States. Children with PACS1 frequently exhibit similar facial features. Kelly's extreme developmental delays include her inability to speak, problems with motor skills, low muscle tone, digestion issues, ocular abnormalities, and slow growth. Nothing cheers Kelly up like SpongeBob and her twin sister, Sabrina.

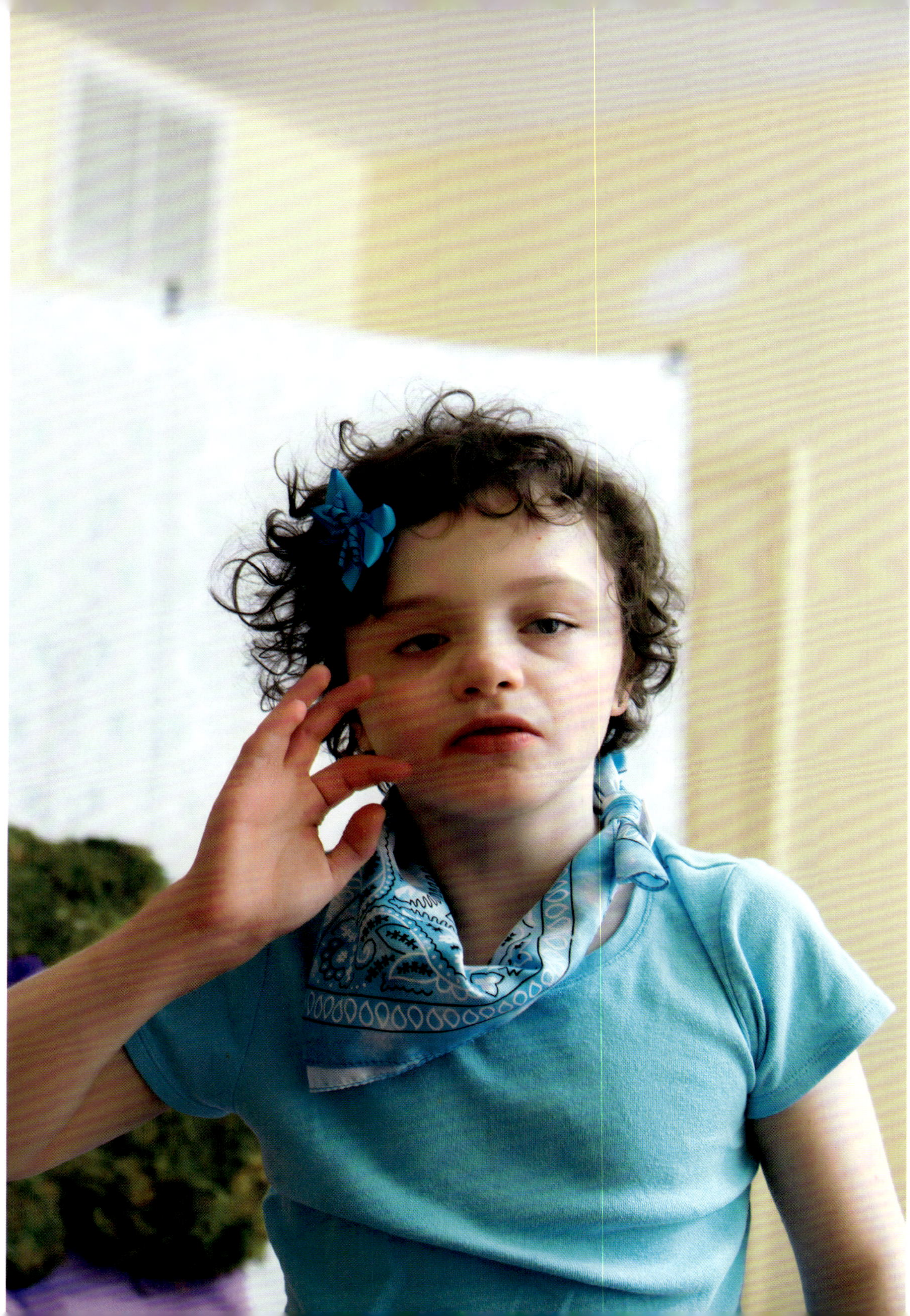

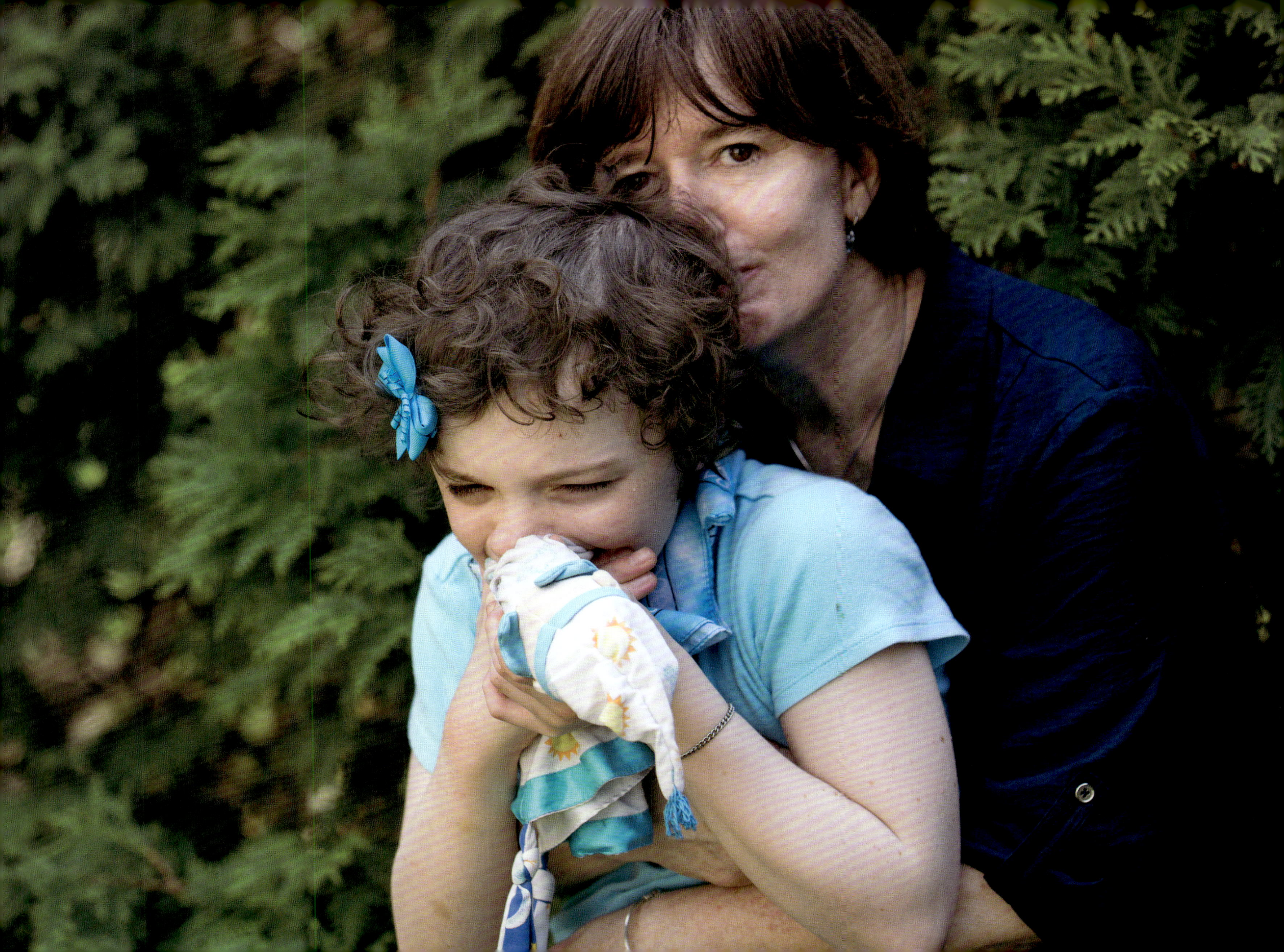

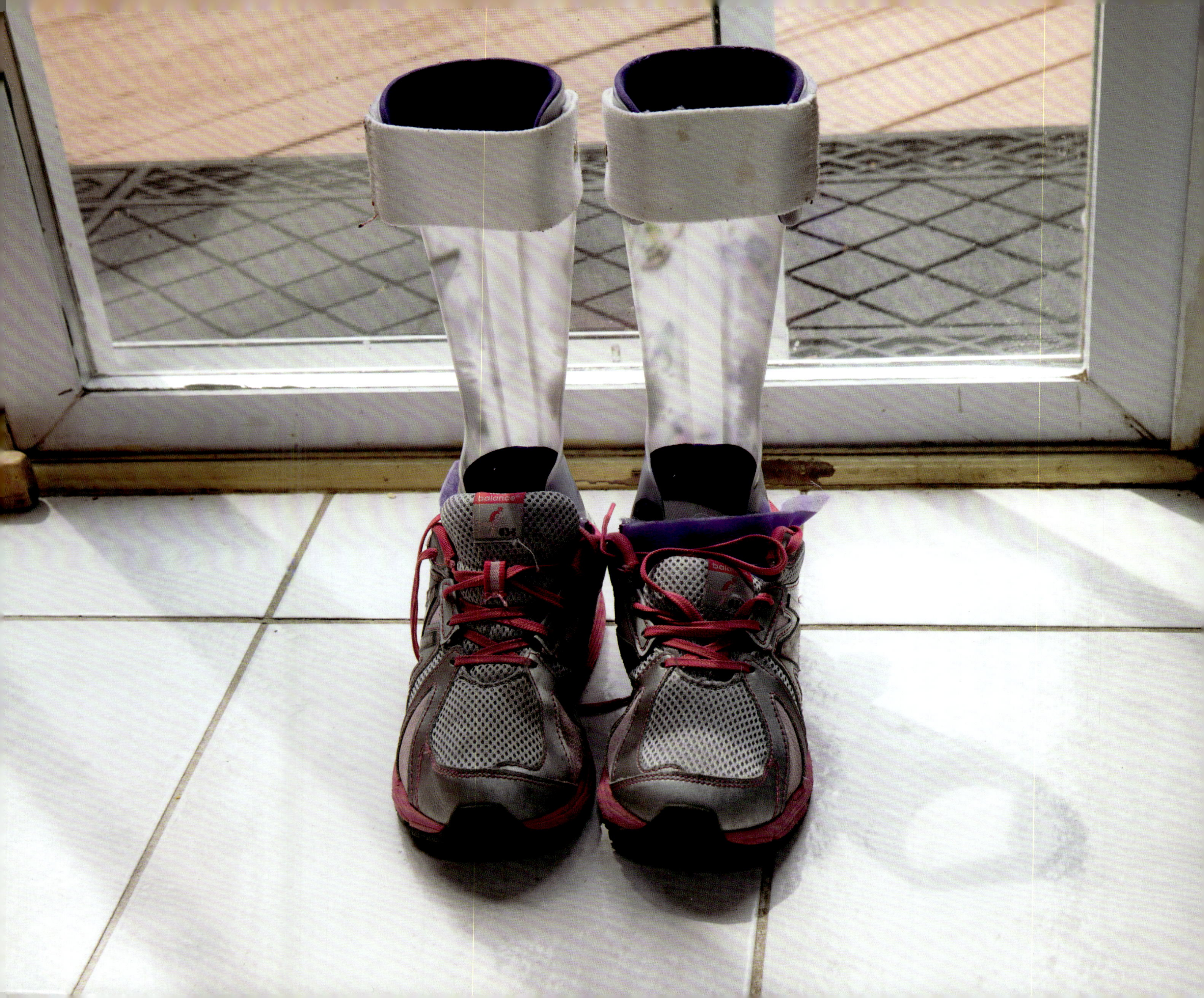
balance

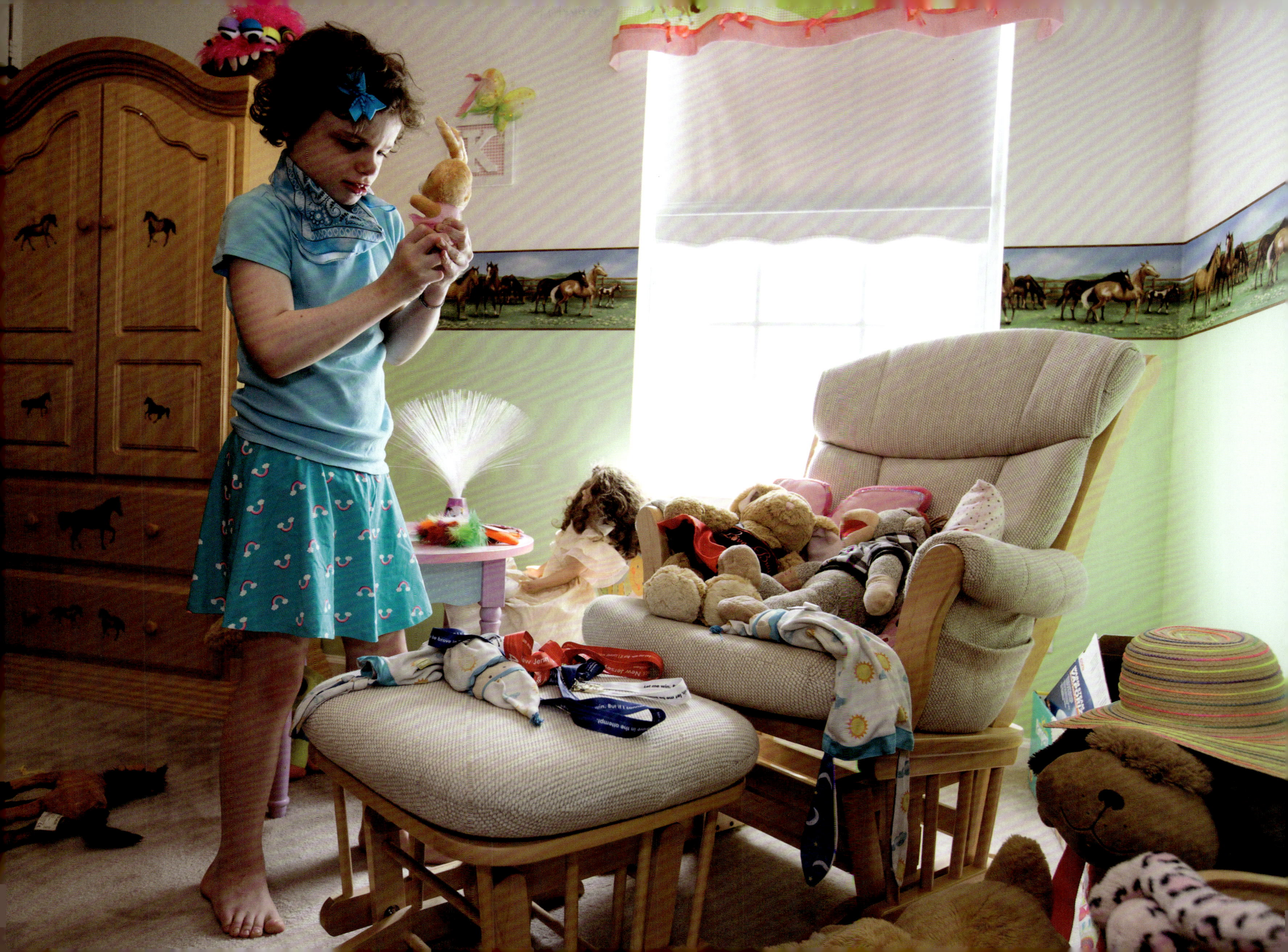

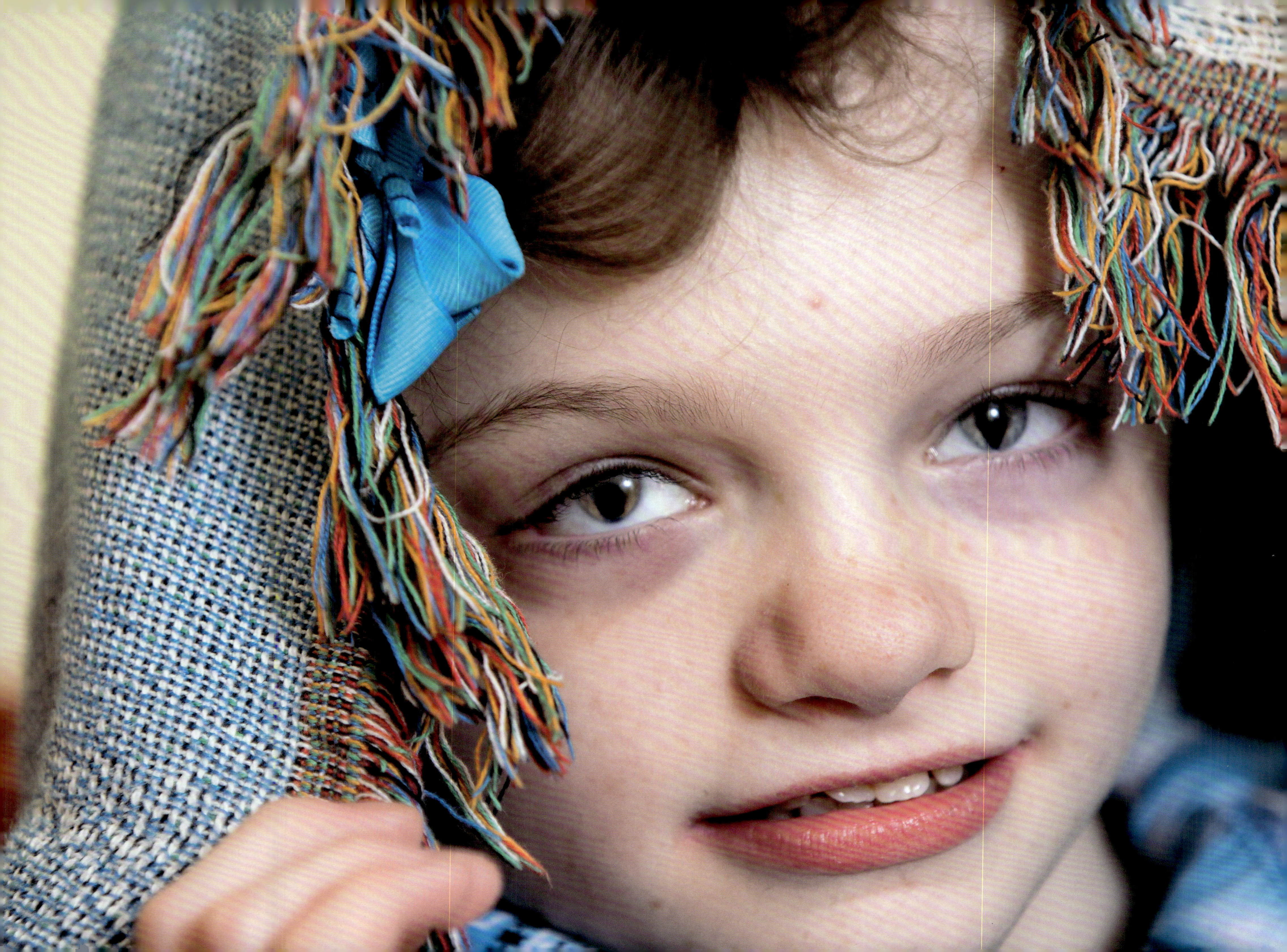

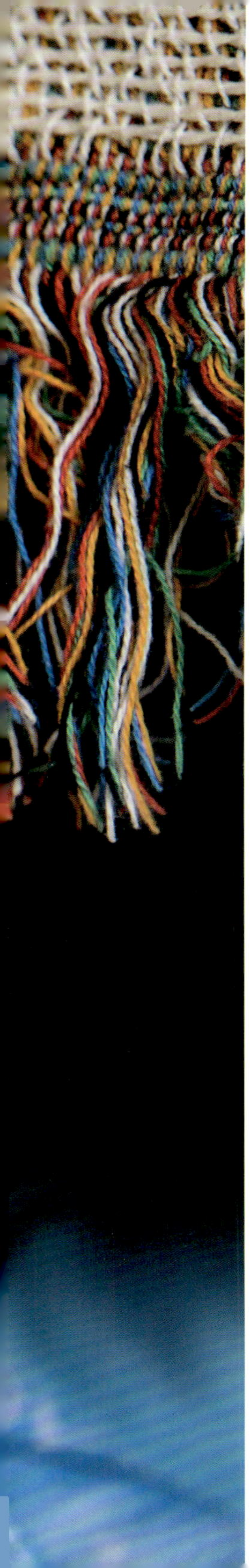

That's what you do with a special needs kid. If you don't have an answer, you treat their symptoms and make them as happy as they can be; give them as much education as you can and get them to progress, no matter what it's called.
– Elizabeth, Kelly's mother

I fix things for a living, and I'm very good at it, and I can't fix this.
– Lief, Kelly's father

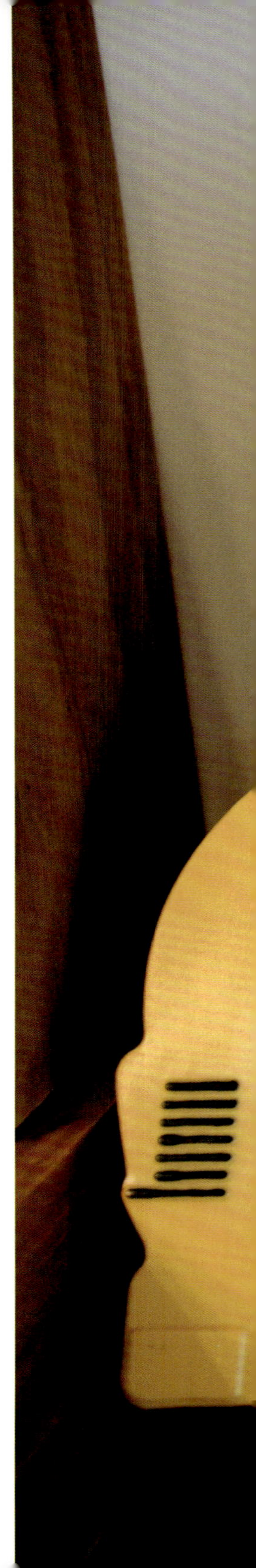

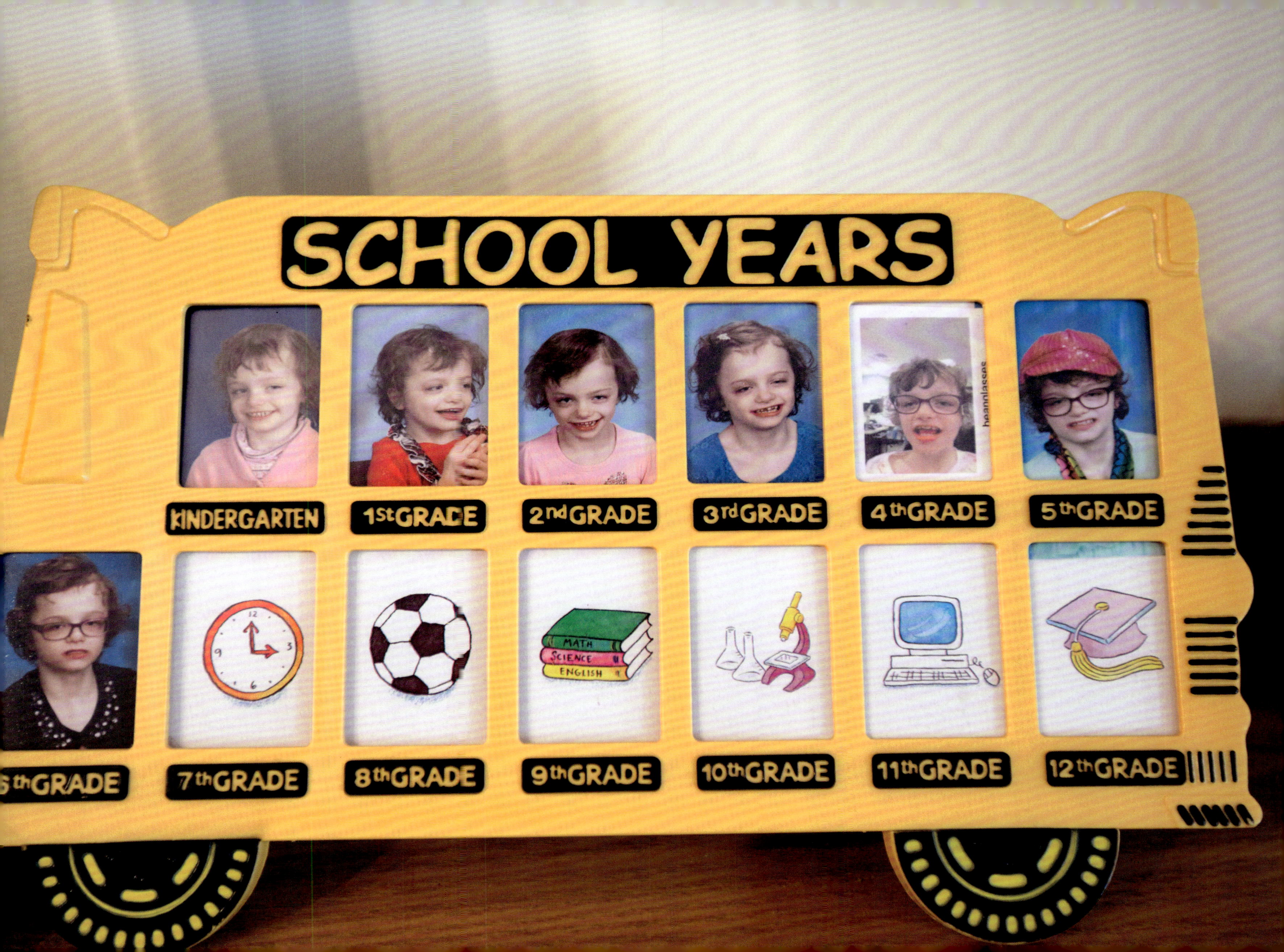
SCHOOL YEARS
KINDERGARTEN
1st GRADE
2nd GRADE
3rd GRADE
4th GRADE
5th GRADE
6th GRADE
7th GRADE
8th GRADE
9th GRADE
10th GRADE
11th GRADE
12th GRADE
MATH
SCIENCE
ENGLISH

Ava

Ava, 8, is one of approximately 50 children in the world known to have SATB2-associated syndrome. It took 6 years to get her diagnosis. There is currently one doctor researching the condition. Ava is nonverbal with no functional means of communicating. She also has severe overcrowding of her teeth, poor fine motor skills, limited receptive language, and low muscle tone, especially in her face, which causes drooling. Ava's doctors do not believe she will ever be able to speak. Despite these conditions, Ava loves riding her adaptive bike, swimming, and running, and is always smiling.

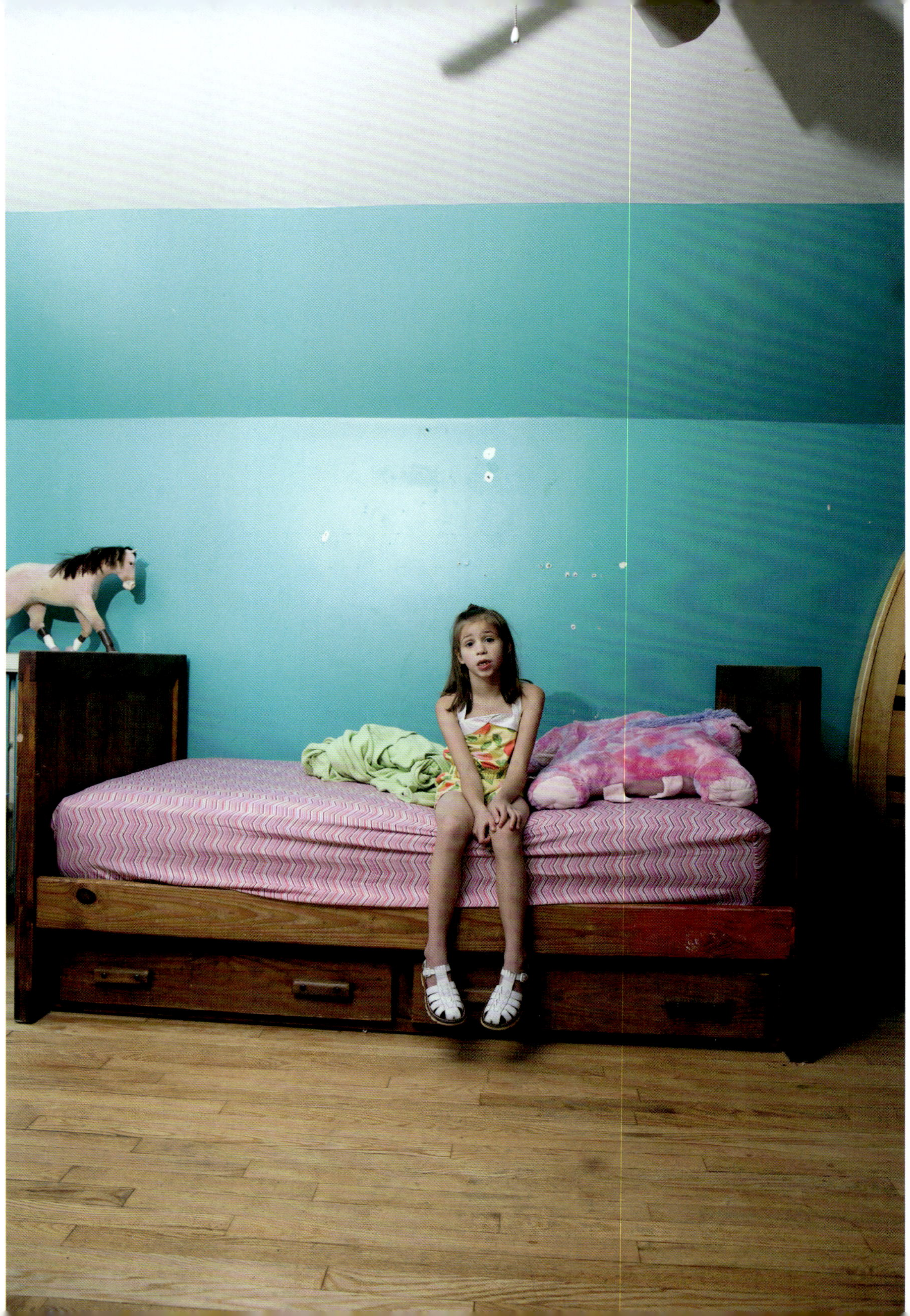

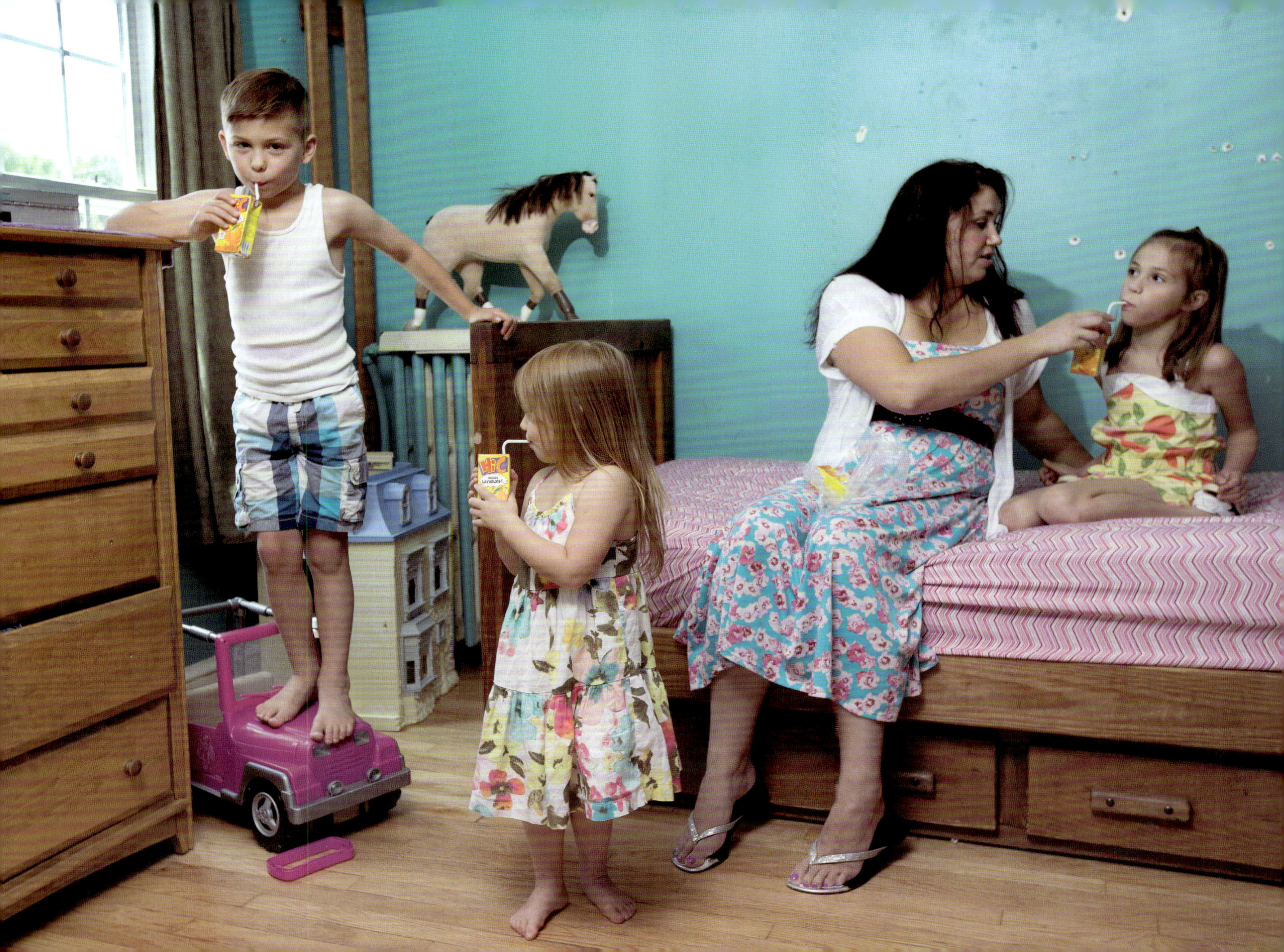
Hi-C
LAVABURST

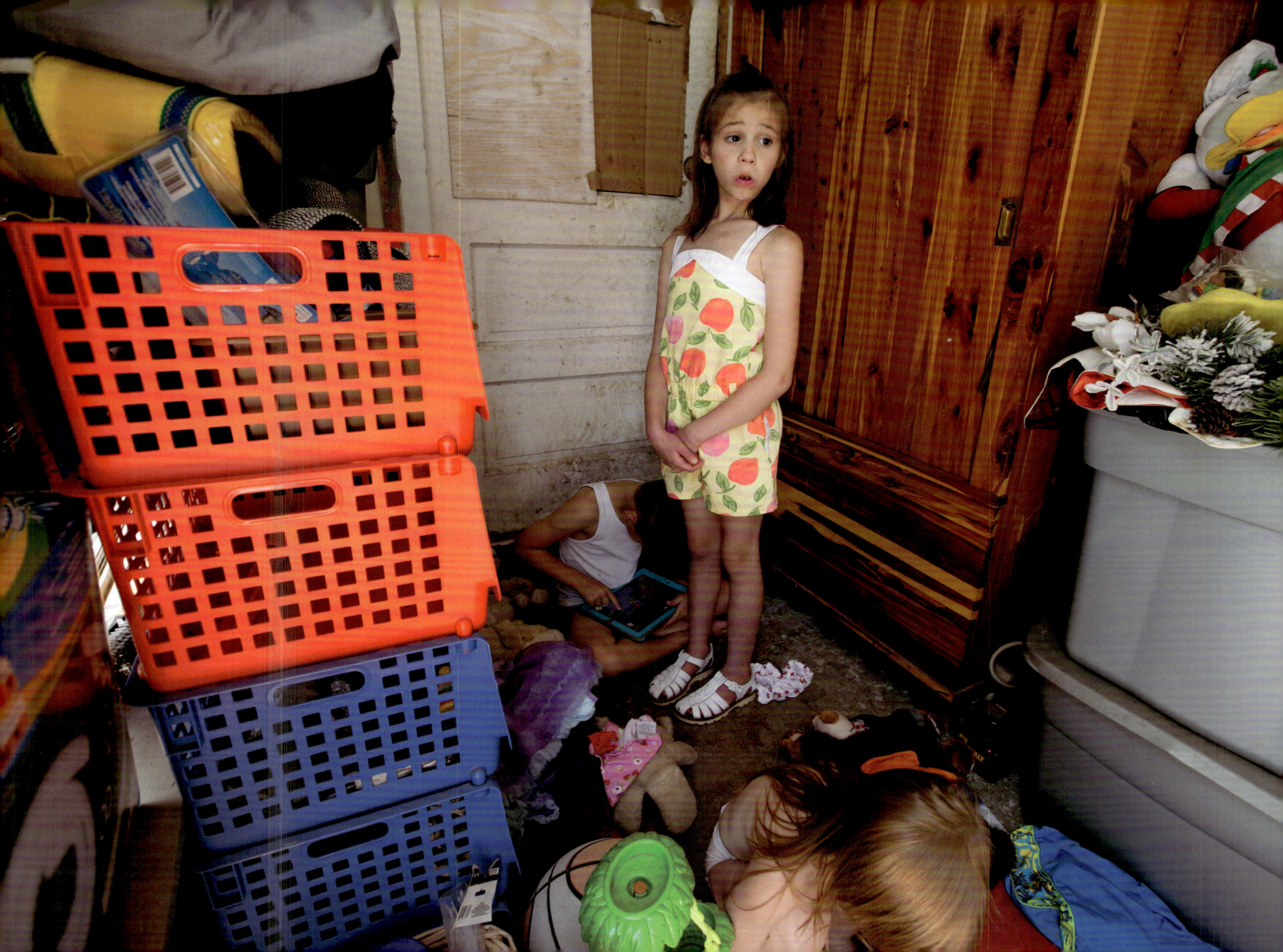

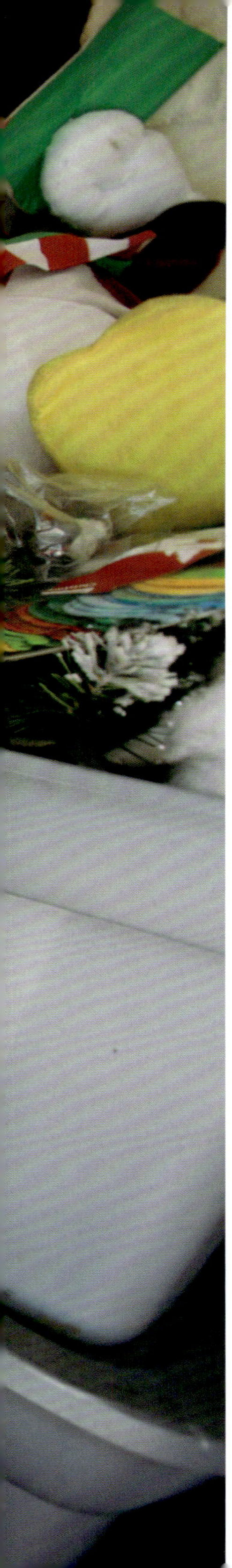

They had told me really early on that they probably would never know exactly what was causing the delays and why she wasn't speaking. I had come to terms with that, I had accepted it. It was hard, it was very hard to come to terms with that and there were days where I would just not leave the house. – Jennifer, Ava's mother

I'm trying to juggle the 3 of them and she's essentially an 18-month-old in an 8-year-old's body. If you think an 18-month-old is a little hard to control, put them in an 8-year-old's body. It's really hard.
– Jennifer, Ava's mother

You look at her and you think she's typical, and she's not. There's a lot that goes along with it. Trying to do anything as a family is hard. Trying to take them out anywhere because people look at her and they expect certain things and it's not the way it's going to happen.
– Jennifer, Ava's mother

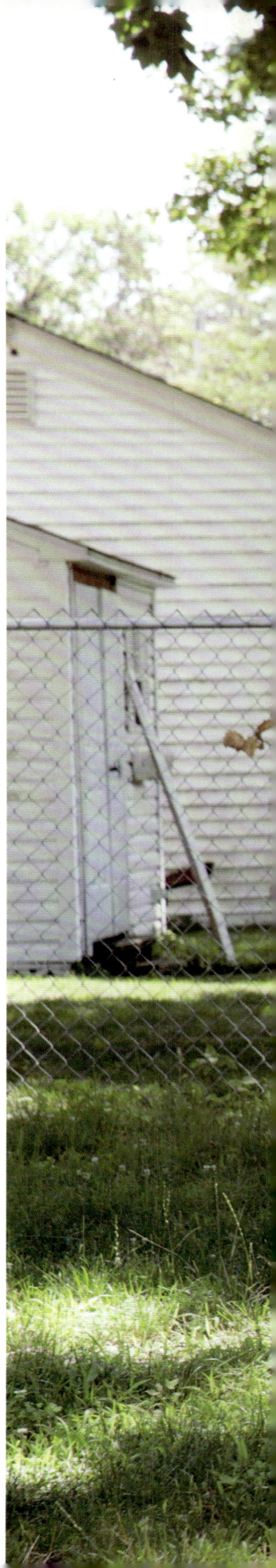

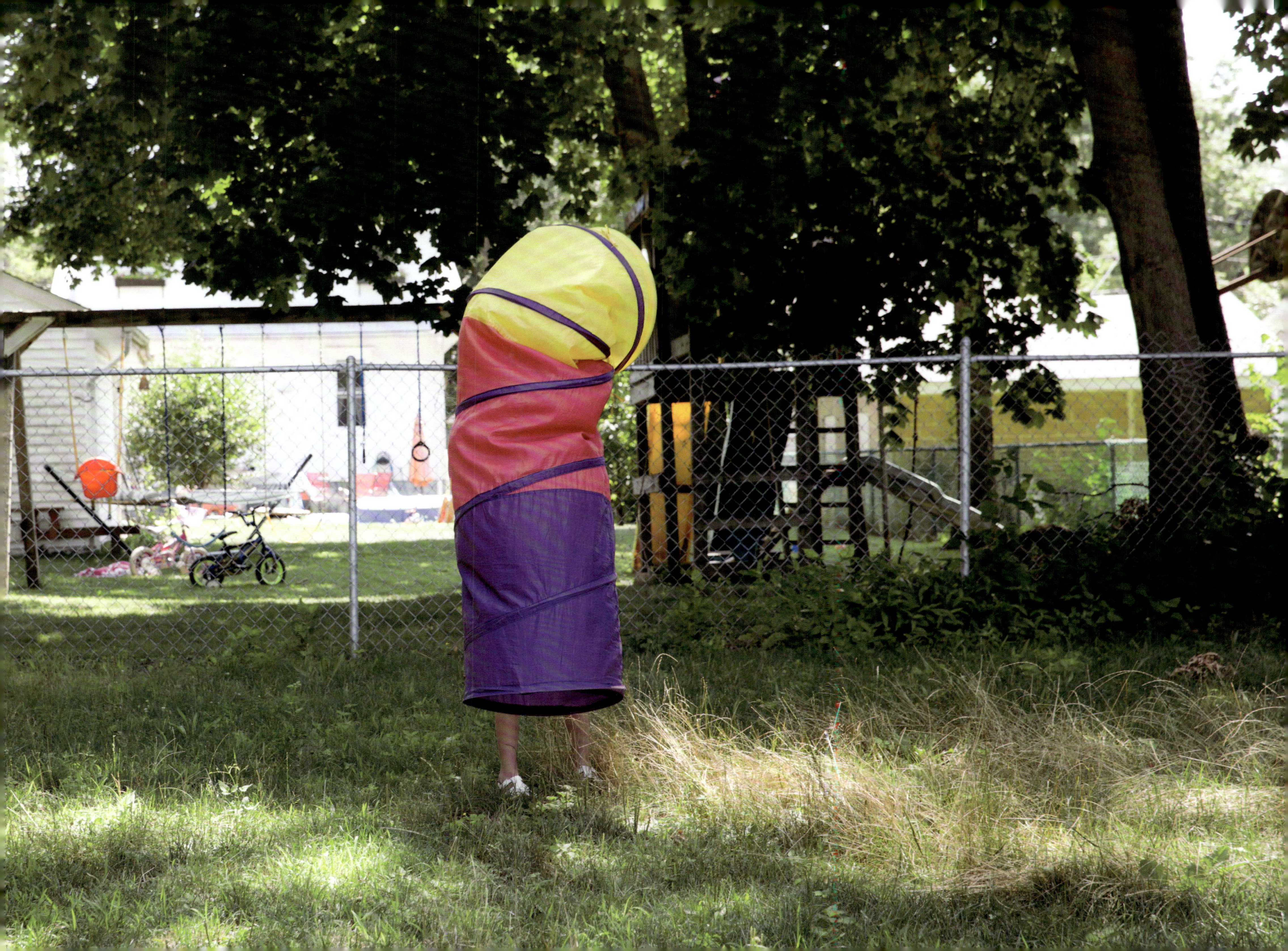

LEFT: MACKENZIE IS PUT IN A SPECIAL STANDING CHAIR THAT KEEPS HER UPRIGHT SO SHE CAN STRETCH HER MUSCLES.

RIGHT: THIS MACHINE CLEARS OUT THE MUCOUS FROM MACKENZIE'S LUNGS.

Mackenzie

After nearly a year of testing, Mackenzie was diagnosed with Tay-Sachs, a terminal genetic disorder that progressively destroys nerve cells in the brain and spinal cord. Before her birth, her father had been genetically tested, but not for all the possible strains of Tay-Sachs—a mistake attributed to either carelessness by doctors and geneticists or the simple fact that health insurance didn't cover the tests.

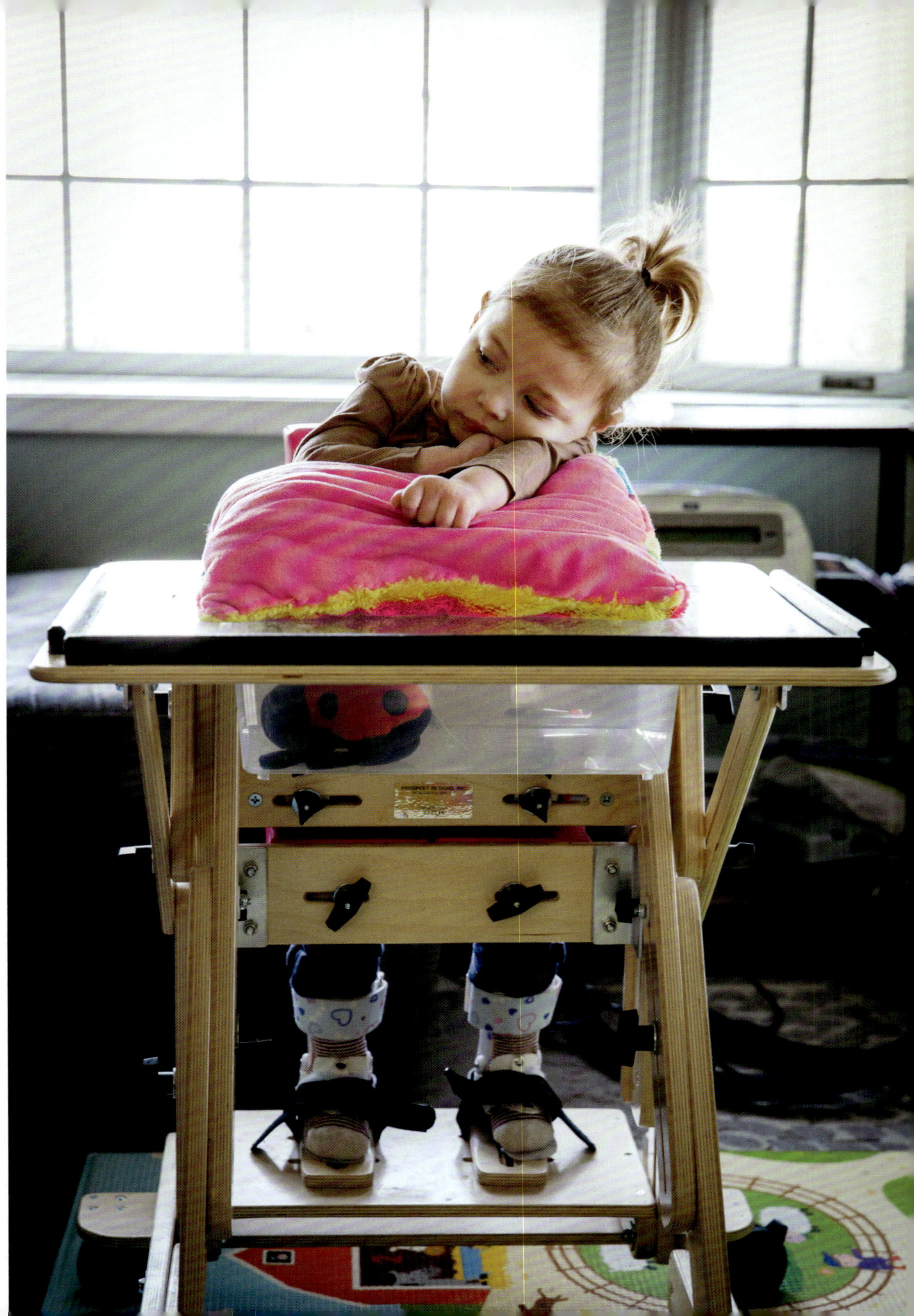

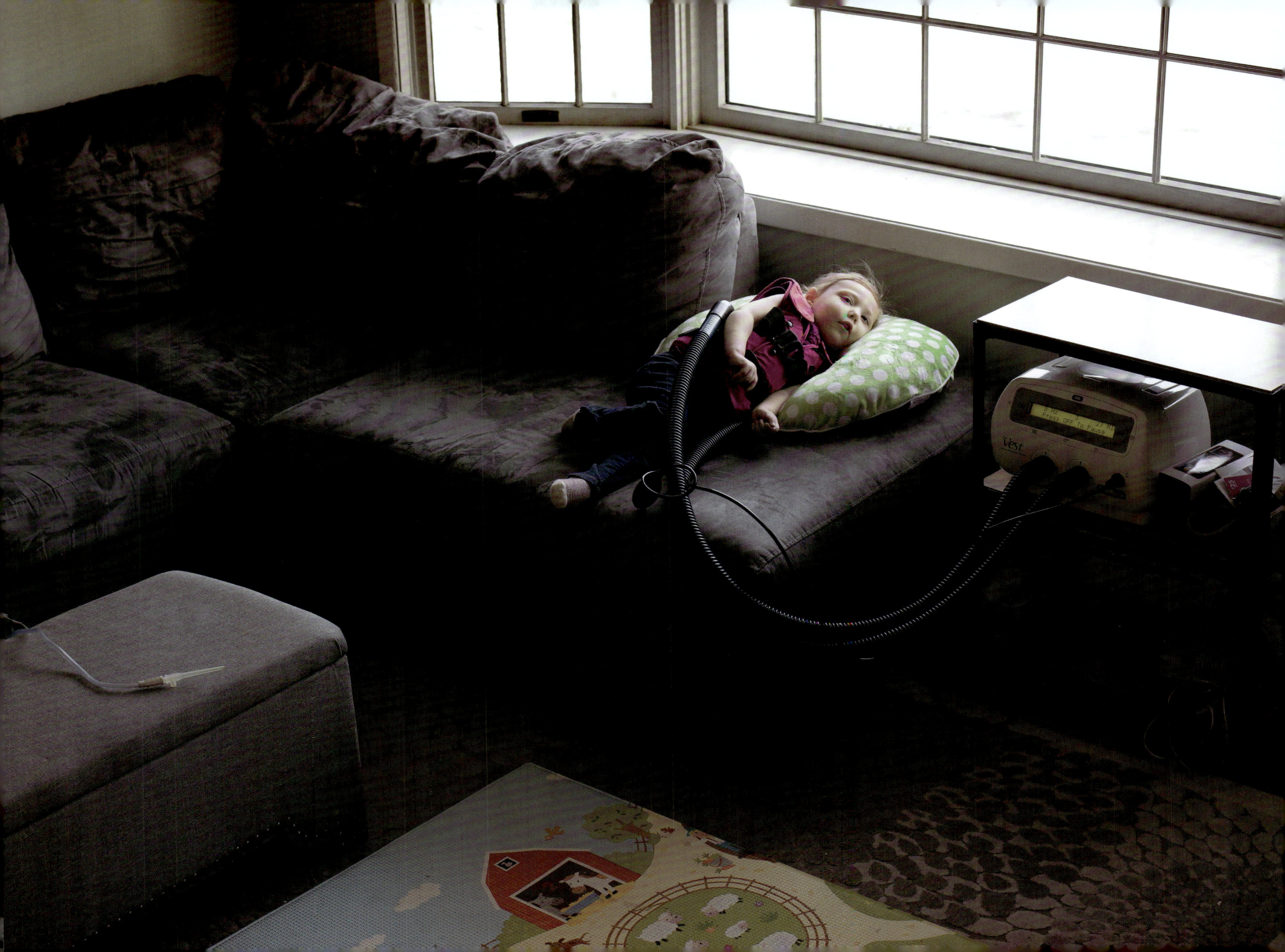
Press OFF To Pause
Vest

When we went to get her diagnosis, our first question was, "But we were already tested for this and why wasn't this caught on the prenatal screenings?" He was a neurologist, so he deferred us to genetics who said, "No test is perfect."
– Colleen, Mackenzie's mom

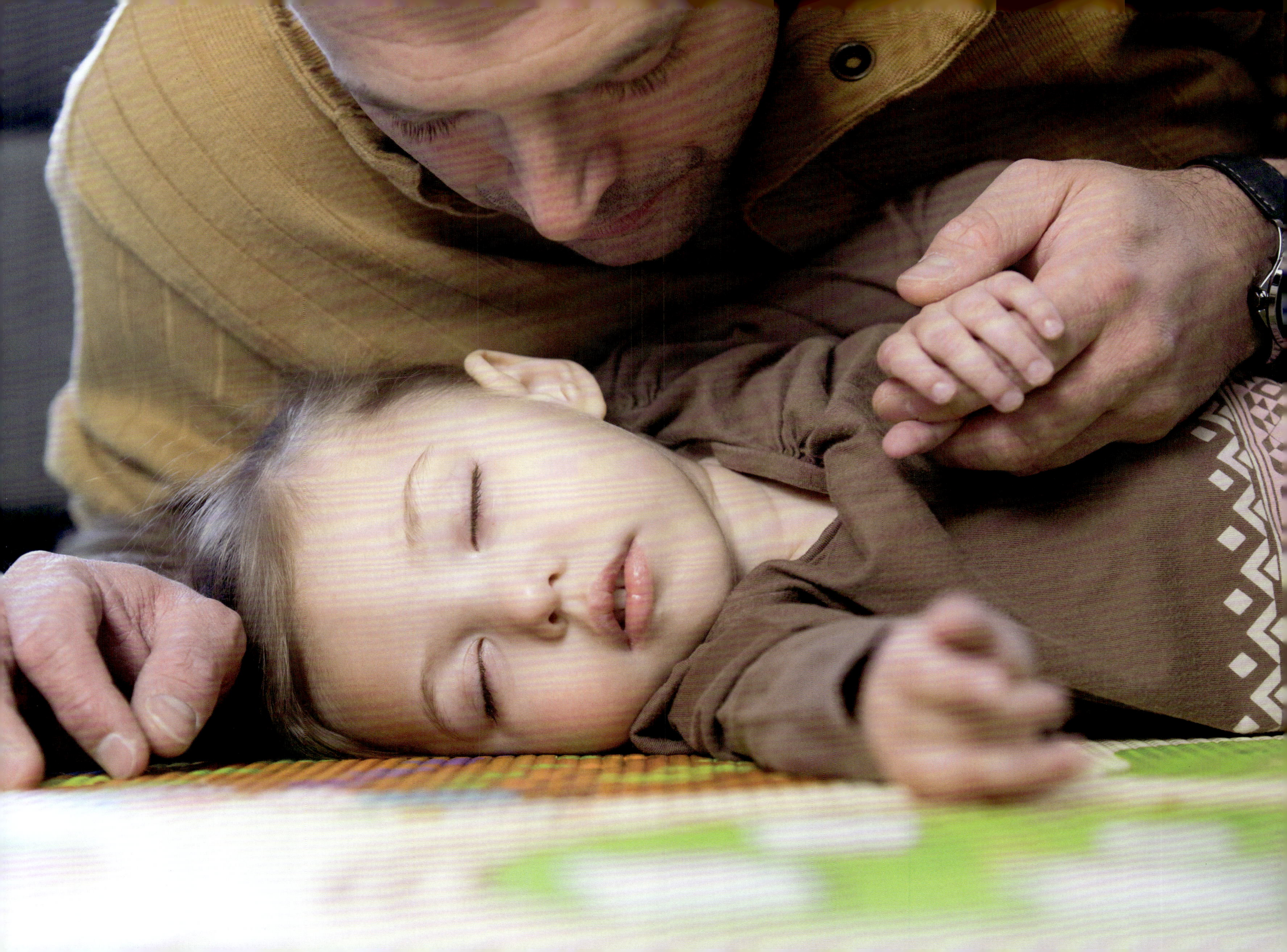

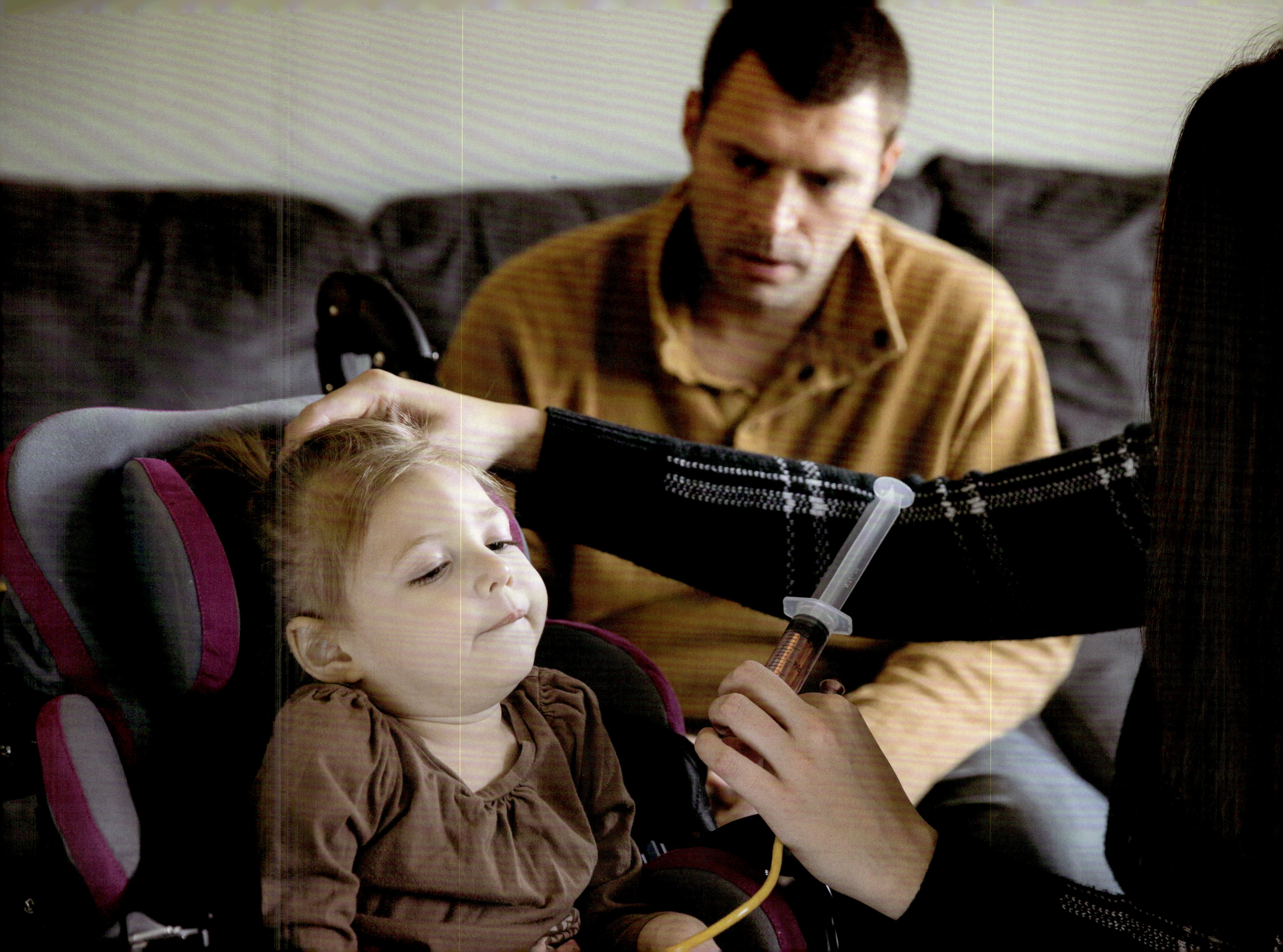

MACKENZIE'S MOM FEEDS HER DAUGHTER SEVERAL TIMES A DAY AND WILL DO SO FOR THE REST OF HER SHORT LIFE.

We try and take everything one day at a time. One day is going to be hard. The next day could be good. We enjoy the good days, remember them, and just don't take anything for granted.
– Brian, Mackenzie's dad

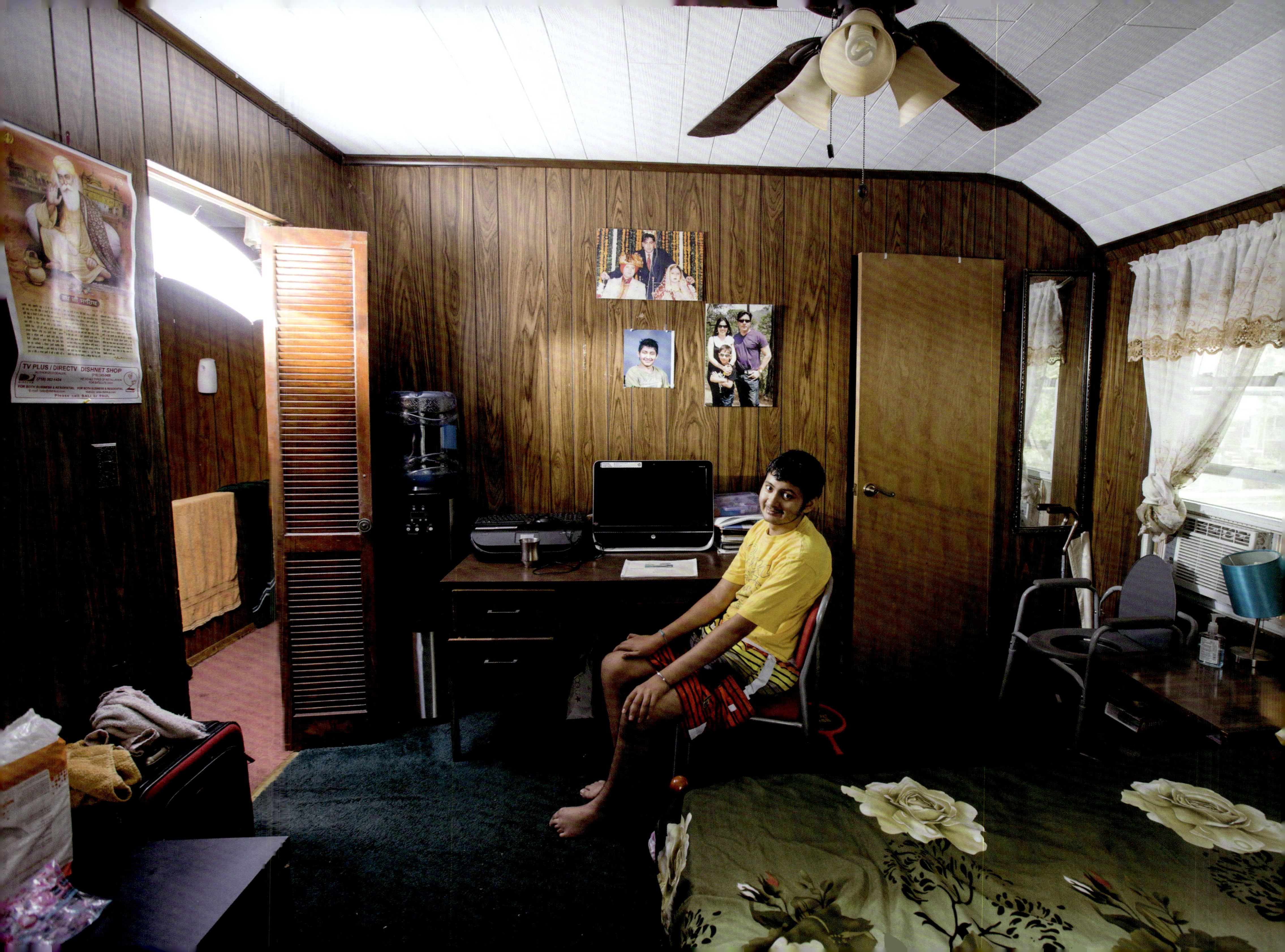
TV PLUS / DIRECTV DISHNET SHOP

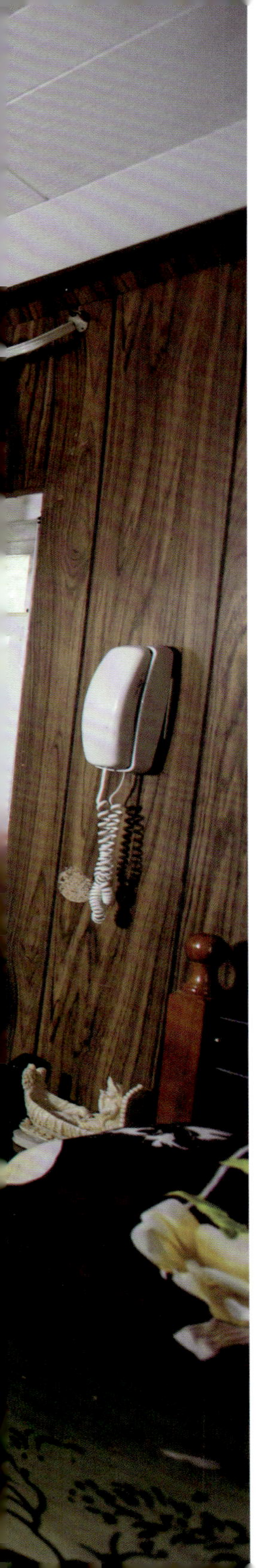

Shaan

At the age of 14, Shaan was medicated for OCD. At 16, he unexpectedly went into cardiac arrest and almost died. Blood work during his recovery revealed a genetic mutation—ALD, X-linked adrenoleukodystrophy—a progressive disease that affects the nervous system and adrenal glands. Though there were no indications of his illness before his teenage years, he now has trouble speaking, listening, and understanding verbal instructions. He is unable to self-feed or take care of himself without assistance. Shaan likes watching TV and playing games on a phone.

He was a normal child. He could do anything, but now, he's in a wheelchair. He cannot walk. We went to school, but he gets therapy and he needs someone all the time with him. It's so hard. He cannot go to college right now because of this. Life is what really changed.
– Ritu, Shaan's mother

We have to do everything. It's not easy. He's just staying home. We have no place; we don't have any information. There's no help. He has no social life, no friends. – Ritu, Shaan's mother

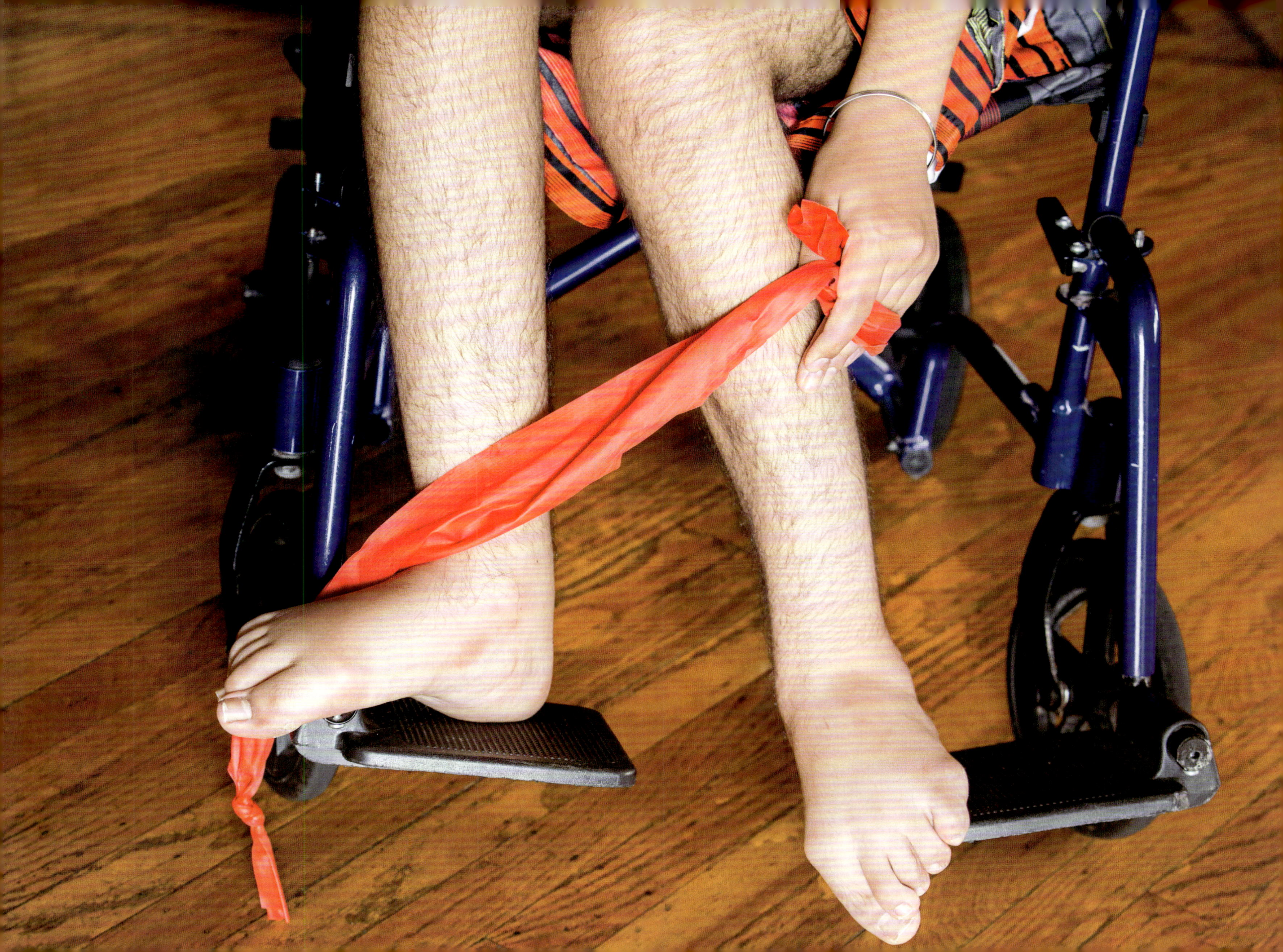

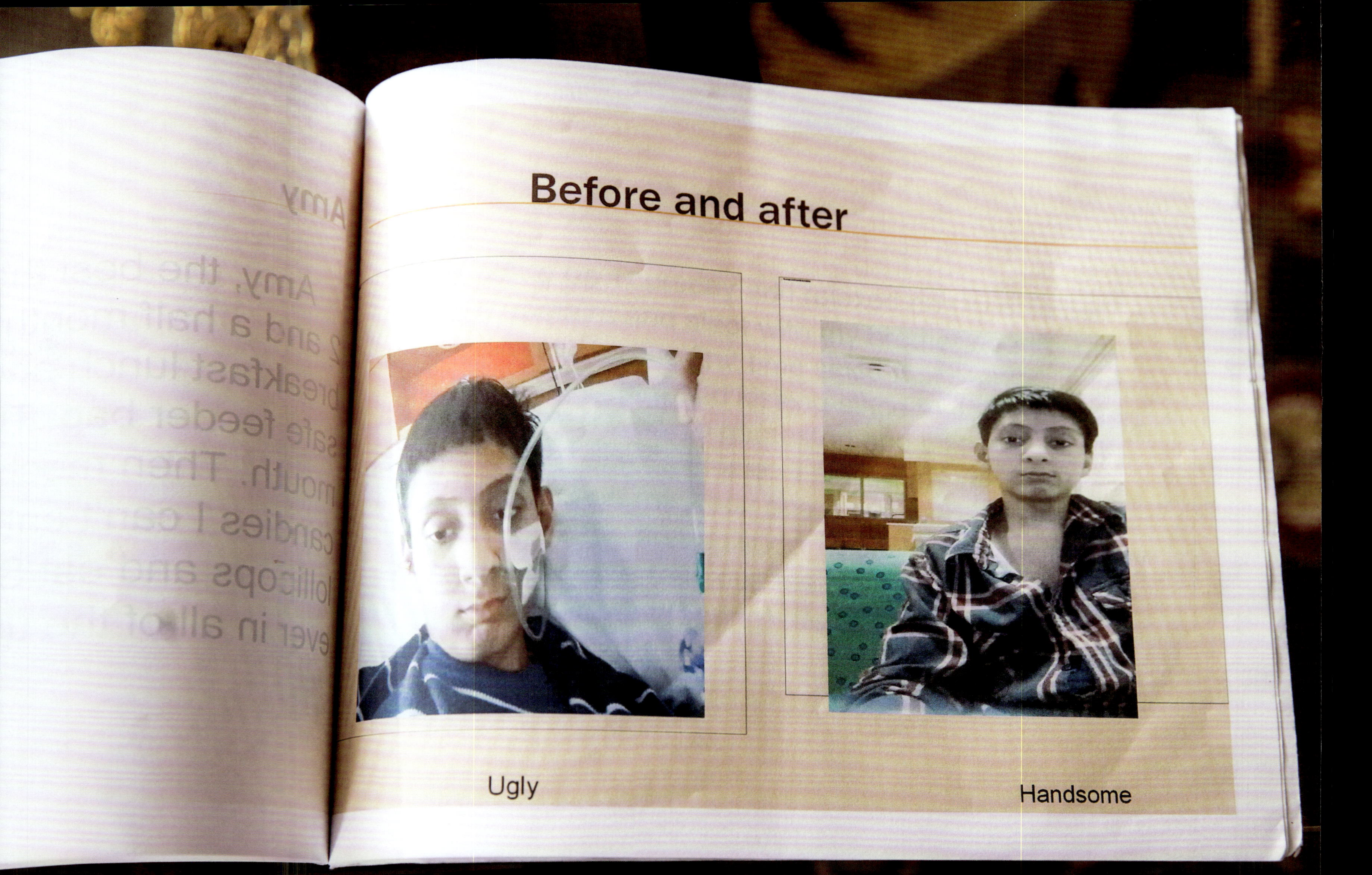
Before and after
Ugly
Handsome

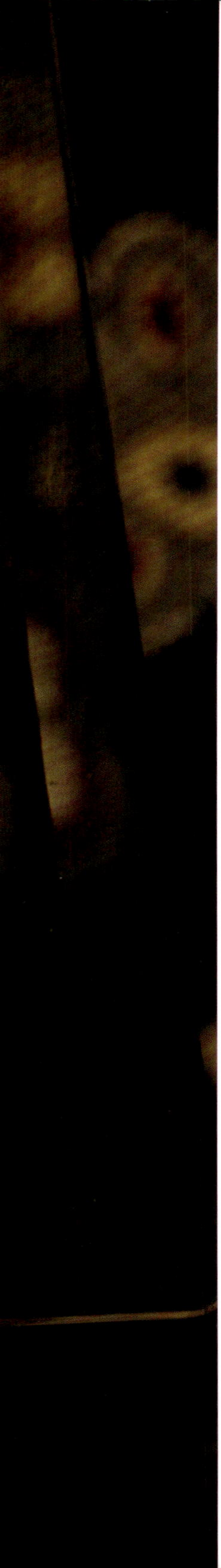

WHILE IN THE REHAB FACILITY, SHAAN CREATED A BOOK WITH HIS LIFE STORY.

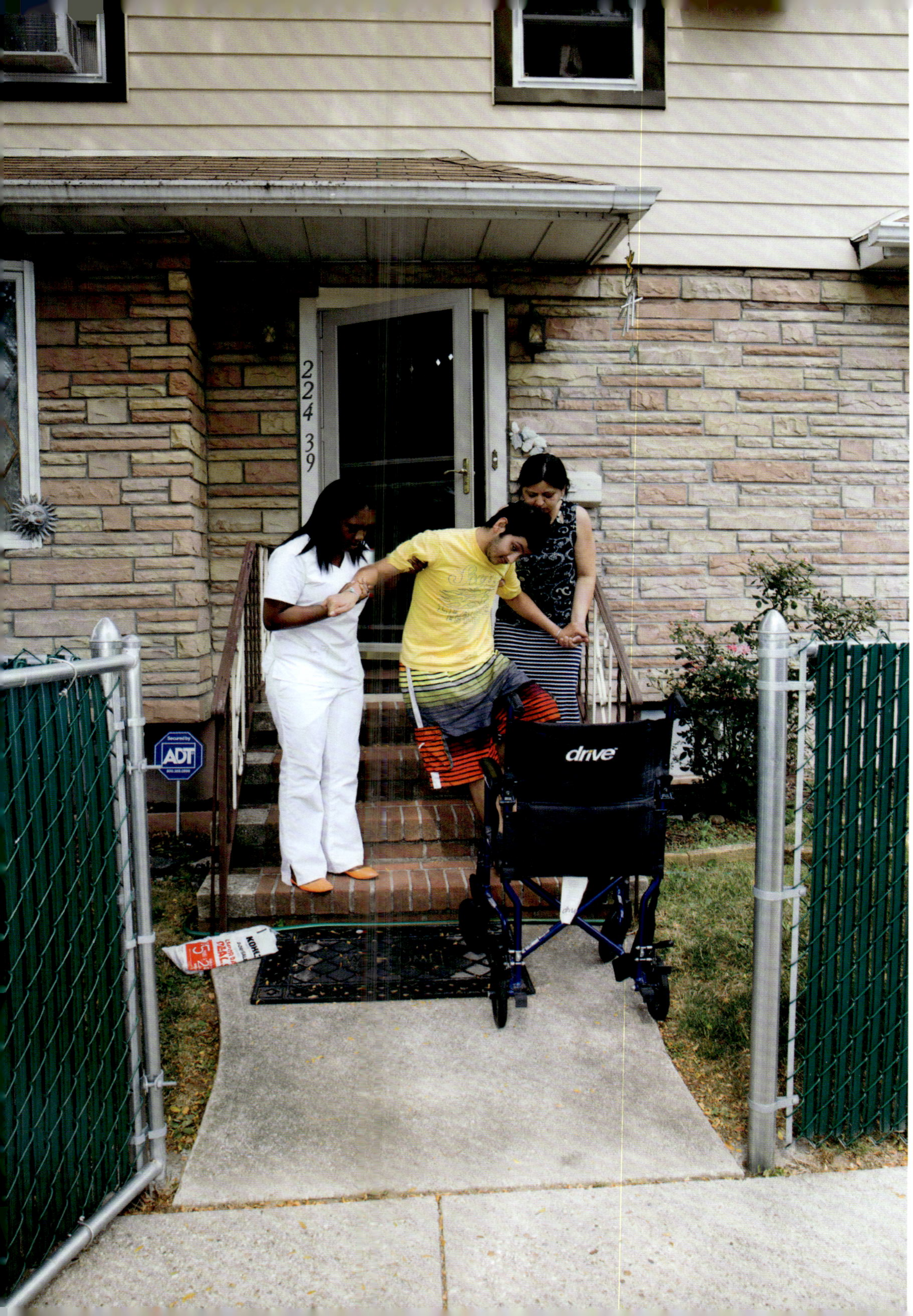

All I want for him is to enjoy his life and for him to feel alive. Whatever he can do, he should be able to do and enjoy. Do something. There should be more facilities for the teenagers who have a disability. They should have more places, more help for them. – Ritu, Shaan's mother

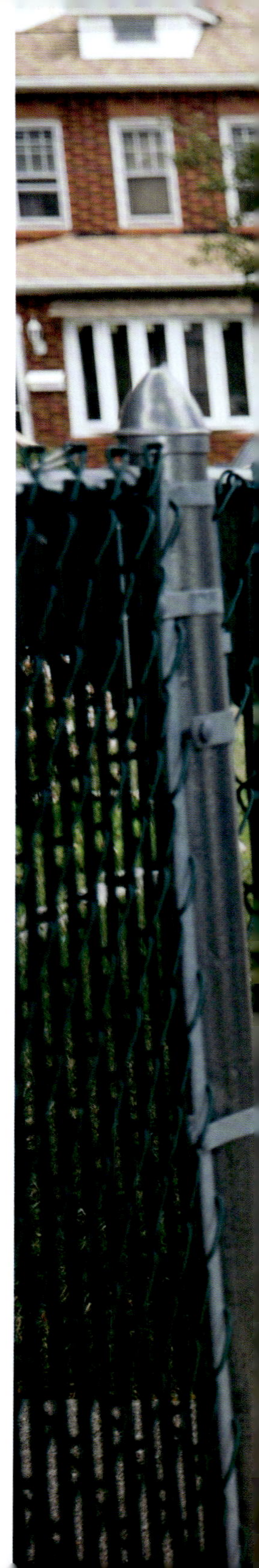

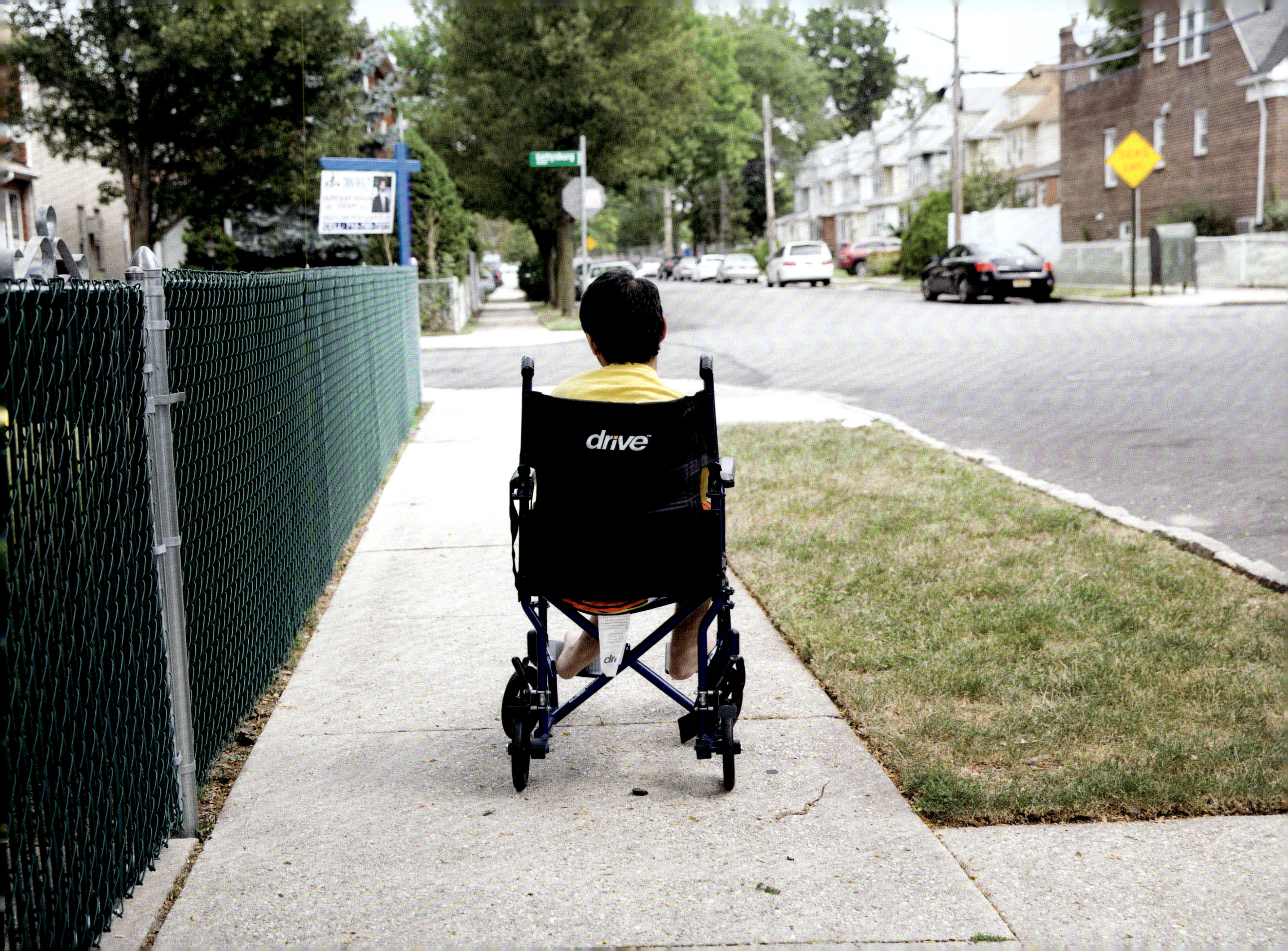
drive

Clara

During a third trimester ultra sound, Clara's parents received the news that their daughter had rhabdomyomas, or benign heart tumors. Clara also has tubers growing in her brain, which cause developmental and language delays. In order to minimize the seizures, the speech center of her brain has been removed.

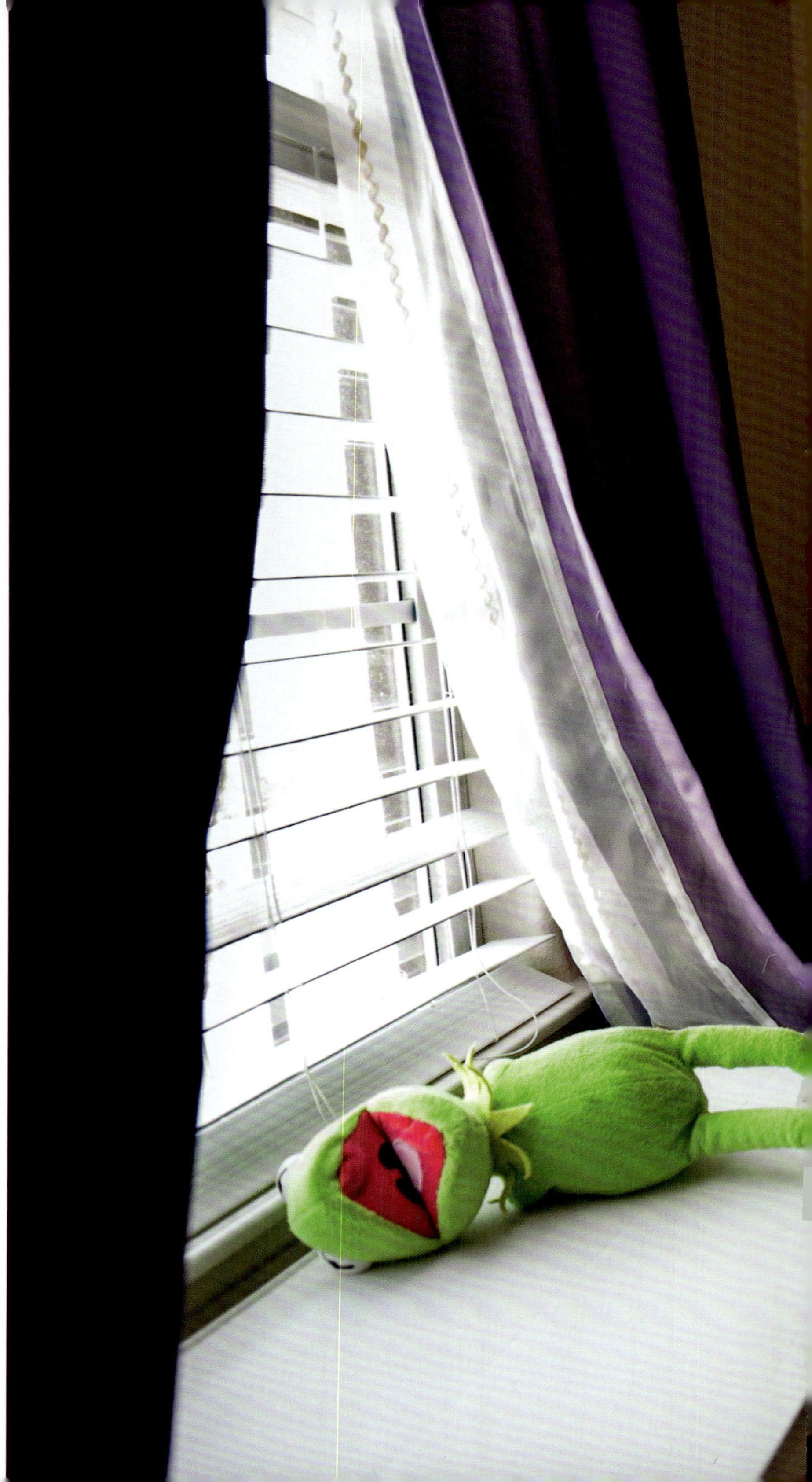

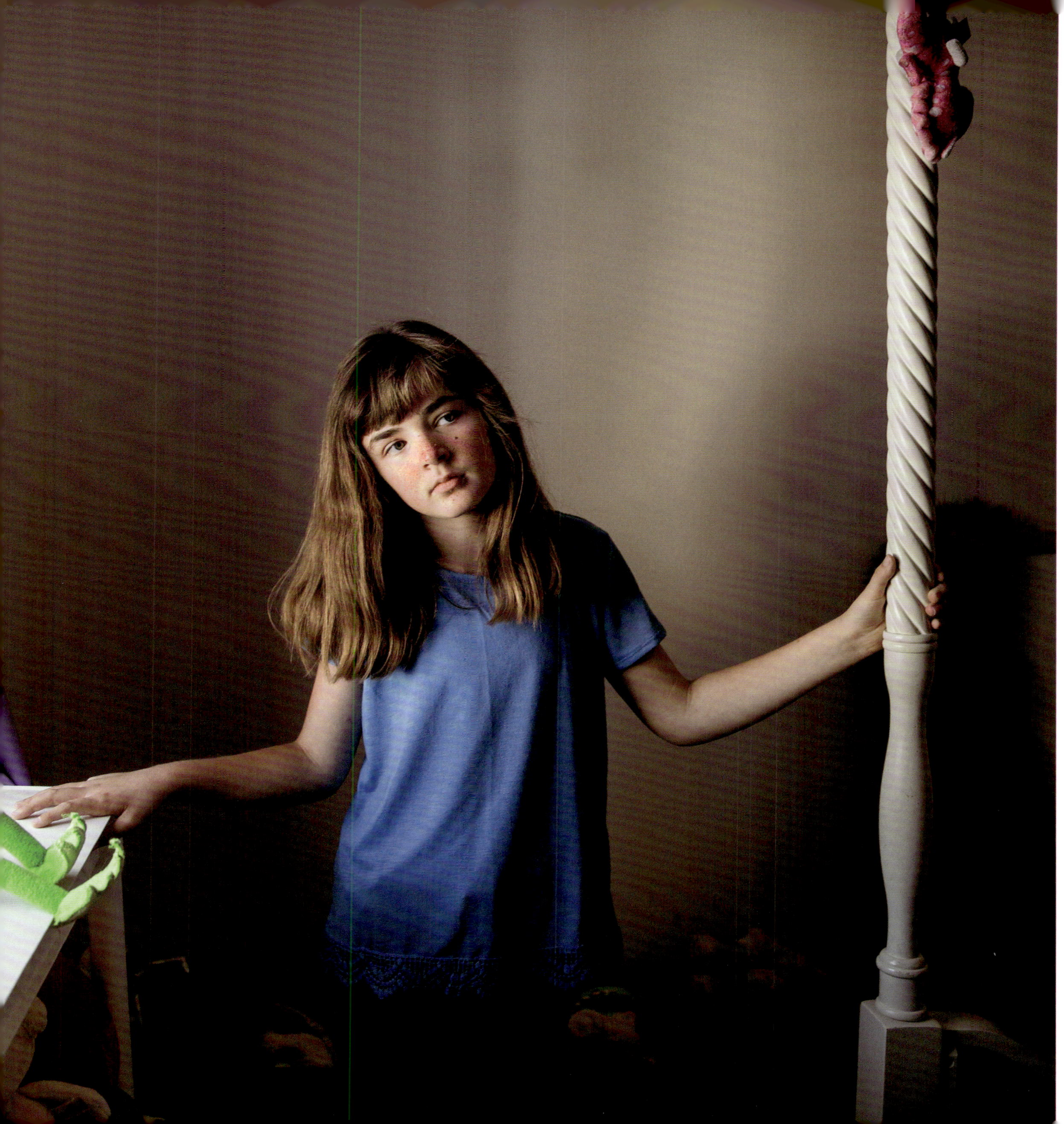

We don't know what her favorite color is, we don't know what her favorite food is, we don't know why or why not she'll do or not do certain things. You know, without that ability to express what she understands, she must feel frustration for that too, and we know that she does get frustrated, a lot.
– Joe, Clara's dad

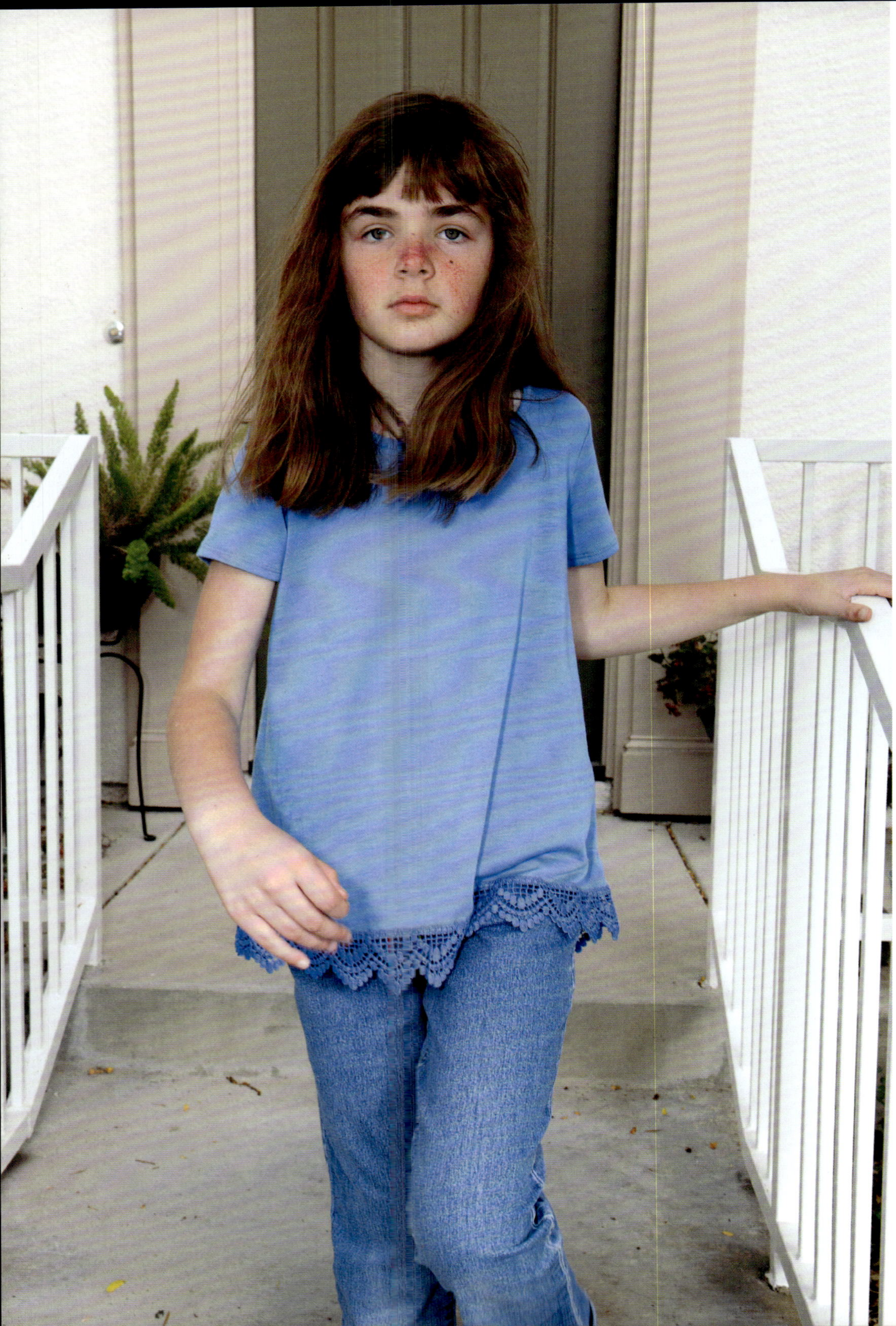

IN ADDITION TO EPILEPSY, AUTISM, AND TUMORS ON HER FACE, KIDNEY, AND BRAIN, CLARA HAS SCOLIOSIS.

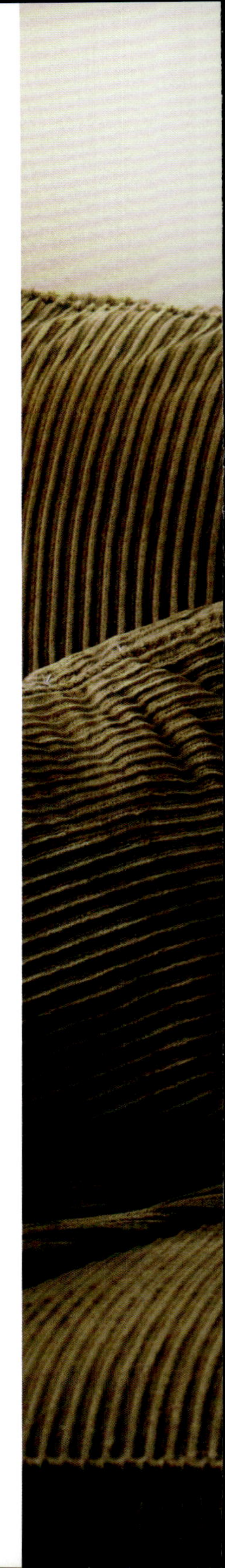

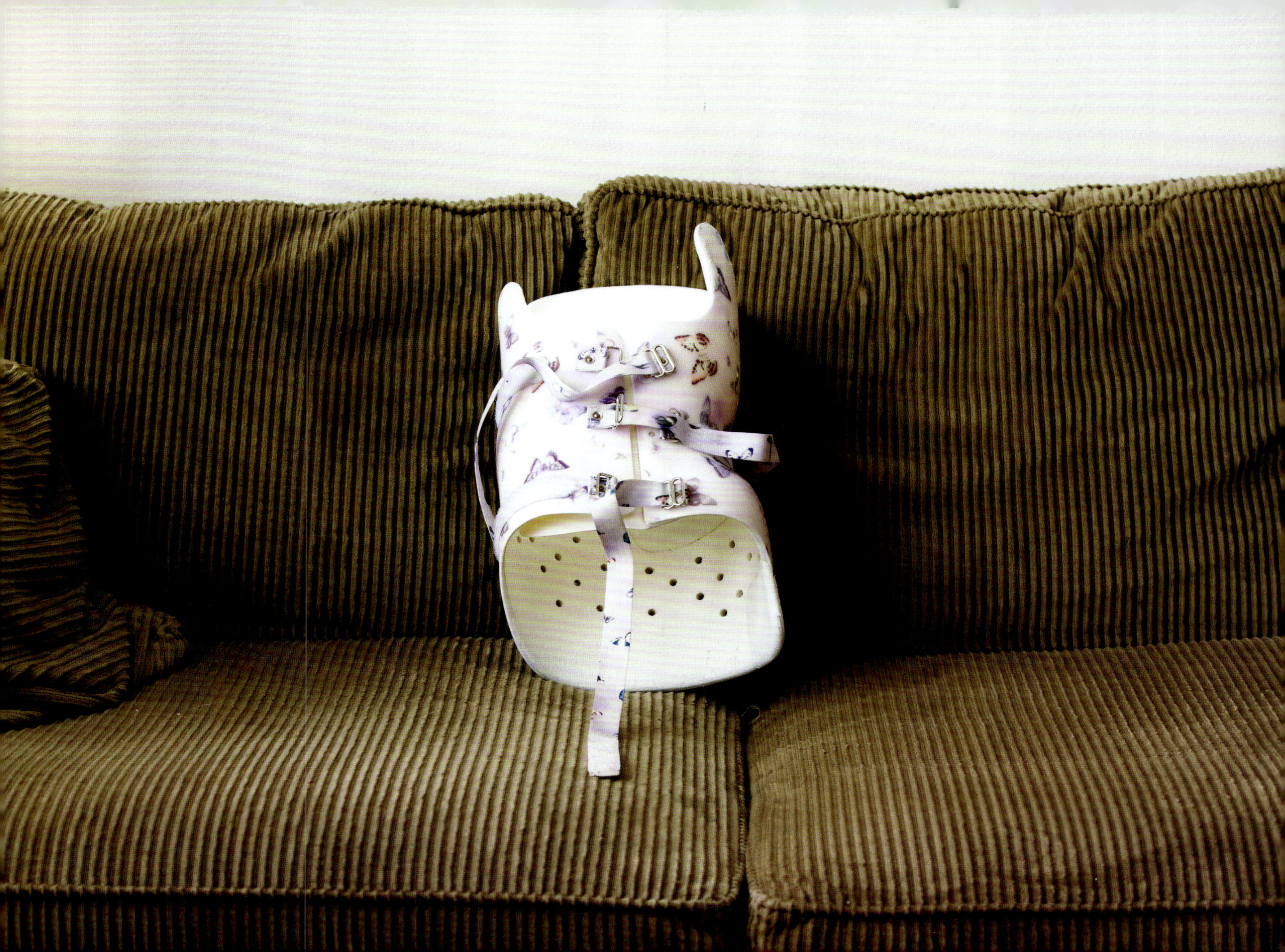

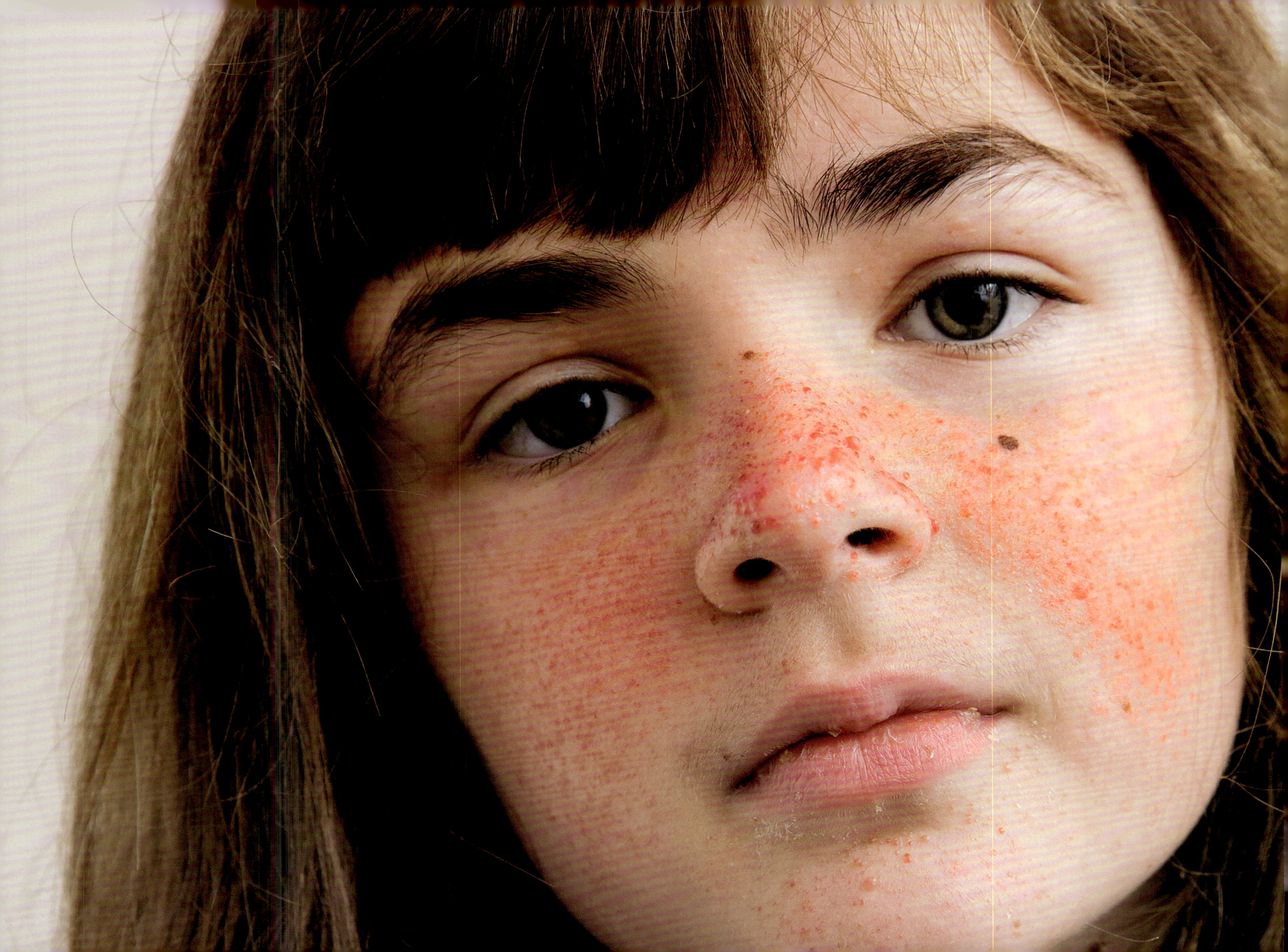

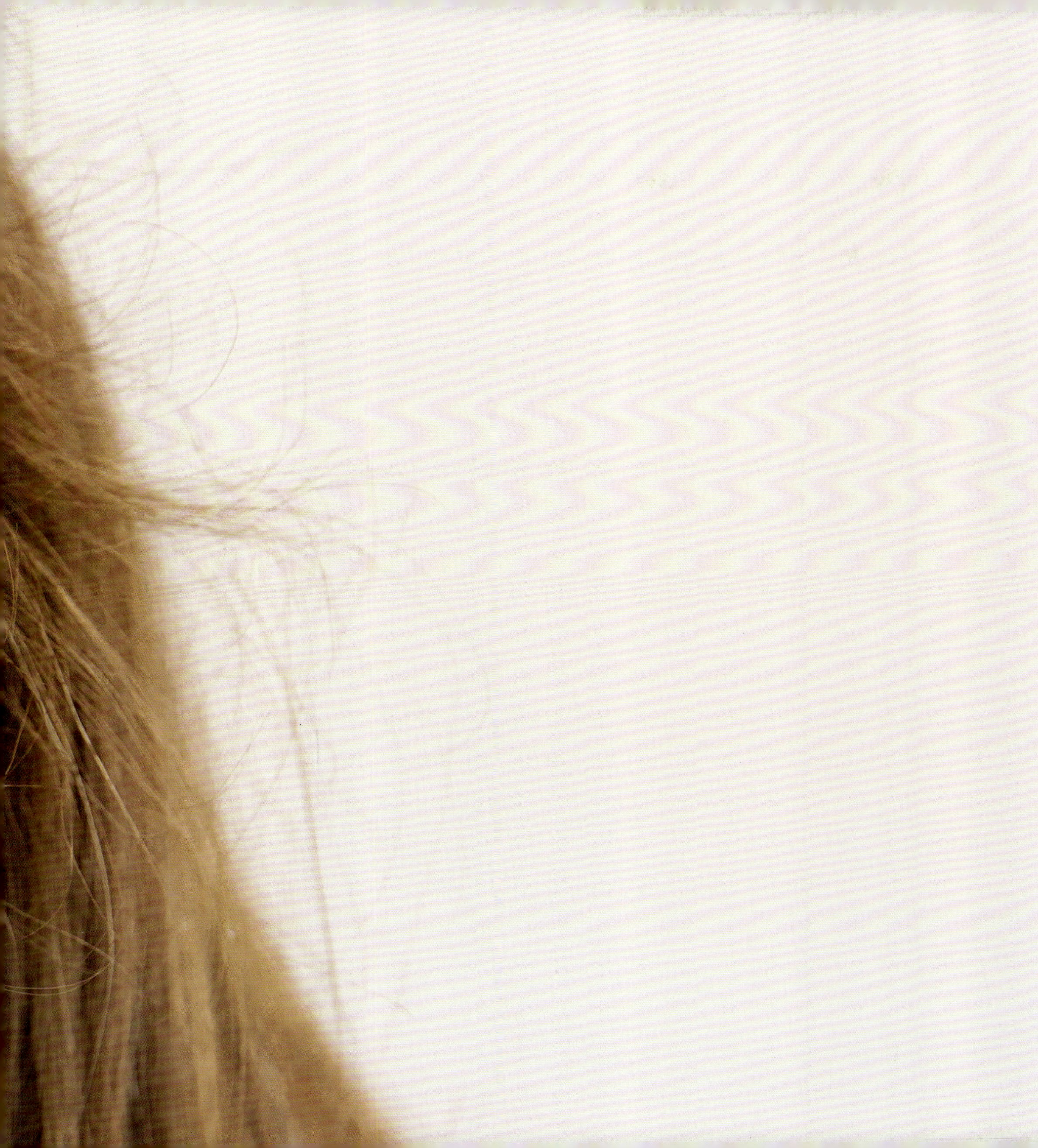

She's in there. There's so much more going on than we can see. Once you clue into that and you start to see those moments, it makes it much easier to overcome the depression and the lack of expectation of her ever being something, because you know, there's more in there when you see those moments. It gives you hope and happiness. – Joe, Clara's dad

Acknowledgements

This book would not have been possible without the support of so many.

First and foremost, I would like to thank all of the families who welcomed me into their worlds and allowed me to document their beautiful children and unique stories. All of you radiate perseverance, patience, and perspective. I admire you deeply.

To my extraordinary husband Bob and my children Maya and Liam, who gave me the freedom to sink my heart and soul into this project: Coming home after a shoot always reminds me what is most important in my life, and you guys are it!

To my parents who lived through losing a child to Tay-Sachs disease: You are my inspiration. Your faith in me is immeasurable and means everything. Thank you for believing in me.

I'd also like to thank the following people:

Orly Wiseman for being my voice of reason and celebrating all of my accomplishments.

Ari Haberberg and Jordan Pavlin for always supporting me.

Aunt Dee Dee for consistently being in my corner since I was an hour old.

Stephanie Katzman for reassuring me that families like yours would want to be a part of my project. You are, and have always been, my confidante.

Amyliz Pera for brainstorming for hours with me that day in June until I finally came up with this idea. It ultimately changed my life and I am deeply grateful.

My production team:
Robert Peacock, photo editor. Your discerning eye and expertise was paramount in producing this book.
Monty Pera, designer. You took a very difficult topic and designed an extraordinary book that marries imagery and text so elegantly.
Heather Slingerland, photography assistant. Thank you for accompanying me on those long car rides. Even though we skipped meals and worked for hours, you always kept smiling.
Jude Tan, photo assistant. Thank you for traveling to LA.
Ricki Harris, text editor. Your talent goes way beyond your years.
Susan Ciccotti, copy editor extraordinaire!
Ed Wiseman, Kickstarter video editor. Your work is always emotionally charged and simply beautiful.
Ari Haberberg, Kickstarter videographer. Thanks for putting up with me as the "talent" and keeping me from crying on camera.

I'd like to thank the following people for their generous contribution:
The Brock Family
Jocelyn and Paul Silverman
Gili & Benjamin Haberberg
Sid Dugar
The Charmak Family
The Berke Family
The Katzman Family
Dan Rafalin,
AvroKO Hospitality Group
Megan Weston
Michael Fennelly
Ross Martin
Hill Country Barbecue
Doori Chung
Kerry Heffernan
Josh Even
Dakota Shy Vineyards
Todd Thaler
Greenblatt & Agulnick, PC
Anthony Milanese
Danielle Lentine & Mark Schultz
Ellen Turchyn
Claire & Cliff Kahn
Abby Lagunoff
Jennifer Brown
Ari Haberberg & Jordan Pavlin
Barrie Gillies & Bill Drummy
Rafi Farber
Jill & Arnold Weiss
Neil Jacobson
Donna and David Providenti
Ronald Brown
Jennifer, Brian, Madison and Gavin Greene
Jadwiga Jesionowski
Sylvia & Al Ades
Lynn Lievense

David Seiden & Cyndi Sterne
Jeff & Barb Seiden
Eric Messinger
Elon Bezner
Bary & Rosy Bezner
Meg Whitbeck
The Hansen Family
Shelly & David Mitnik
Erika Rachel
Debby Stone
Janine Rosen
Howard Cooperman
Stella Chang
Betty Katz
Brenda Adesso-Frounfelker
Carol Hall
Melissa Spillane
Elizabeth Breden
Naomi Jacobson
Teri Tsang Barrett
Lauren Domitrovits
The Berger Family
Donna Barklage
The Wiseman Family
Nikki & Brad Silver
Jason Denmark
Jackie & Seamus Delaney
Scott Edelstein
Albert Kalbfleisch
Erika Millet
Jamie Kogod Levin

Erin Peter
Alisa Stein
Asher Mendelsohn
Kate Callery
Leonard Majzlin
Daria Royzman
Rachel Honickman
The Chow Family
Dina Ortner
Deborah Carlson
Nora Speer
Megan Weston
Laurie Waddell
Wendy Halperin
Brenda Wilensky
Nicole Johnson
Lauren Feldman
Jessica Rakshys
Shari Abercrombie
Kenneth V. Breglio
Carol & John Leiggi
Josh Fenton
Francois Krygier
Mimi and Rick Comerford
Dor & Liat Skuler
Sandra George
Ellis Denmark
Candence Fairbanks
Sanford Hausler
Elissa Campbell
Jill Schulman

Eric Carson
George Taylor
Anne Lenihan
Lori Kravitz
David Greenspun
Paulette Torres
Fighting H.A.R.D. Foundation
Linda Doyle
Grace Koo
Wendy Zajack Lipshultz
Amyliz & Monty Pera
Jeremy & Corey Fox
Michele Rosa
The Santos Family
Edward & Alyssa Seiden
Dana Wancjer
Karen Kogod
Deborah Meyers
Alyson Abramson
Stacy Ezra
Ann Biederman
Barbara Cuttriss
Sharlene Moore
Kimberly Campbell
Traci Kampel
Jeanmarie Lombardi
Lawrence Chen
Seth Borden
Catherina Park
Rebecca Shapiro
Ian Garlic

Patrick Simeone
Lauren & Dave Wiseman
Aleeza Nemirof
Amy Chang
Kyle Osborne
PhotoShelter
Sara Bobertz
Andrew Solomon
Jennifer Rubino
Traci Denmark
Karen Novak
Heidi Krupp
Gina de Mendonca
Pamela Trembow
Darya Lehrich Goldstein
Stephen & Rochelle Seiden
Pat Hughs
Jason Silber
Joseph Smith
Toni Lagunoff
Mark Sarfati
Fighting H.A.R.D
Maya & Liam Seiden
Yoav Litvin

About the Photographer

Karen Haberberg has spent twelve years as a professional photographer documenting stories of human resilience: the memories of a Holocaust survivor, the daily life of a developmentally disabled young adult working on a farm, and more recently, kids with rare genetic conditions. Karen's parents lost their first child, Rafi, at age three; he died of Tay–Sachs disease before Karen was born. The memory of the child who died so young is never far from the family's collective consciousness, and inspired the work on this project.

Karen is a New York City based lifestyle and portrait photographer. In addition to her freelance work, Karen lectures and teaches at New York University, the 92Y and the JCC in Manhattan.

For nearly a decade, she served as the Director of Photography and Digital Media at the Jewish Community Center in Manhattan, where she spearheaded photography related programming for children and adults. Karen has also curated numerous exhibitions and collaborated with well-known photographers such as Annie Leibovitz, Elliot Erwitt, Joyce Tenneson, Gillian Laub, Bruce Davidson, among others.

Her photography has been shown in numerous gallery exhibitions, magazines and newspapers including the New York Times, The Wall Street Journal, The Daily News, Huffington Post, Time Out NY, Daily Mail, Cosmopolitan, New York Family Magazine, Forbes, and Fit Pregnancy. Her work has been featured on ABC News and NY1.

Karen holds a BA from Brandeis University and earned her MA in Fine Art and Photography from the ICP. She lives in Manhattan with her husband and two children Maya and Liam.

karenhaberberg.com

Index

An Ordinary Day:
Kids with Rare Genetic Conditions

Published in the United States by
powerHouse Books,
a division of powerHouse Cultural Entertainment, Inc.
28 Adams Street, Brooklyn, NY 11201-1021
telephone 212.604.9074
e-mail: info@powerHouseBooks.com
website: www.powerHouseBooks.com

First edition, 2017

Library of Congress Control Number:
2017946119

ISBN 978-1-57687-861-3

Designed by Monty Pera

Printing and binding by Midas Printing, Inc., China

10 9 8 7 6 5 4 3 2 1

Printed and bound in China

you can build confidence
once you free yourself of
other people's judgements.

nd there was
no way
to avoid the
Cruelness of
the Spinning
Earth.

·Adva
·Don'
·mot

"I'm Fine."
she said.
and she smiled.

you only hate
the road when
you're missing home

I used to
It's funny

Tell me exactly,
in what way
their opinions
matter?

H.O.P.E
Hold on, Pain Ends.

my life was full of Choices,
and you were my [illegible]t
one.

ove is like a
oller coaster.
ou keep spinning
nd spinning and
ventually you want
to throw up.
-Bella

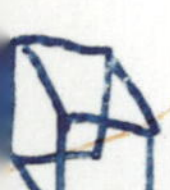

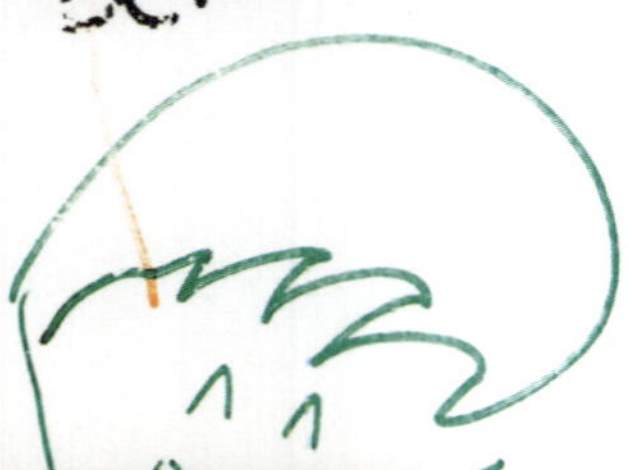

FEAR
has two meanings.
Fear
Face

Breat